Praise for
THE HUMAN SIDE OF CANCER

"For many years Dr. Holland has worked with knowing dedication in an effort to learn from patients struggling with cancer—and the result is a book that tells us not only of the great ordeal those individuals face but also of the wisdom they acquire in the midst of their suffering. Here pioneering psychiatric research and clinical work become something else, something special: a human witness to lives as they unfold with dignity as well as fearful stress."

—Dr. Robert Coles, author of the
Pulitzer Prize–winning *Children of Crisis*

"This book is practical and warm, helpful and with heart, opening new thoughts and ideas while comforting with old-fashioned wisdom. It is a true treasure for cancer patients and their partners."

—Helene G. Brown,
Associate Director, community applications
of research, UCLA Jonsson Comprehensive Cancer Center

"Dr. Holland's book will be of invaluable help to anyone caught up in the saga of cancer—the people who have it, their caregivers, family, and friends. It is a clear, no nonsense, and above all compassionate guide that tells you all the things you wanted to know but were too afraid to ask. Don't go to the doctor without it!"

—Kathleen Chalfant,
actress who starred in the play *Wit*

"Once, Jimmie Holland told me many of these things and made my life more bearable. Now her extraordinary insights are available to everyone—a road map that makes a terrifying journey much less so. She is the bright light in the dark forest, warding off the monsters with wisdom and concern, easing the torture in our minds that comes from the disease in our bodies. If you have cancer, or care for a cancer patient, or simply want to understand how to talk to someone who's been diagnosed, I urge you to read this book. It will change your life."

—Lynn Sherr, ABC News, *20/20*

"Dr Holland, in her inimitable combination of warmth, wisdom, and compassion, speaks out from the printed page. She accompanies the patient and family through the uncharted experience of living with a life-threatening illness in all its facets—the sadness, the uncertainty, the hope. Unlike many books which promise hope through—in her words—'the tyranny of positive thinking,' Dr Holland provides a sense of hope through her profound understanding of the human experience. Any individual or family confronted with cancer will find a gentle and sage companion in this book."

—Barbara M. Sourkes, Ph.D.,
Montreal Children's Hospital / McGill University,
author of *The Deepening Shade: Psychological Aspects of Life-Threatening Illness* and *Armfuls of Time: The Psychological Experience of the Child with a Life-Threatening Illness*

"In *The Human Side of Cancer*, Dr. Jimmie Holland has opened up the black box of emotional turmoil that reverberates in the minds of cancer patients and their families. This pioneer in psycho-oncology also provides helpful guidance in specific techniques of self-empowerment. Importantly, she takes the burden of the disease off the shoulders of the patients. Anyone touched by cancer, personally or in a friend or loved one, should turn for help and comfort to this outstanding distillation of a lifelong professional experience with the emotional repercussions of cancer."

—Sidney J. Winawer, M.D., MACG,
Paul Sherlock Chair in Medicine, Memorial Sloan-Kettering Cancer Center, author of *Healing Lessons*

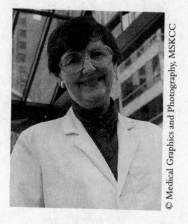

© Medical Graphics and Photography, MSKCC

About the Author

DR. JIMMIE HOLLAND is a recent recipient of the Special Presidential Commendation in recognition of the high quality of her contributions to psychiatry. She is chief of psychiatry at Memorial Sloan-Kettering Cancer Center in New York City, and professor of psychiatry at the Cornell University Medical College. Dr. Holland is the author of the first textbook on psycho-oncology. In 1994 she received the American Cancer Society's highest award, the Medal of Honor. She lives in the New York City area with her husband, James F. Holland, M.D.

SHELDON LEWIS is a journalist specializing in the psychological aspects of health. He lives in New York City with his wife and two sons.

The
HUMAN SIDE
of CANCER

The
HUMAN SIDE
of CANCER

LIVING WITH HOPE,
COPING WITH UNCERTAINTY

Jimmie C. Holland, M.D.,
and
Sheldon Lewis

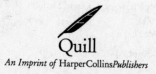

Quill
An Imprint of HarperCollins*Publishers*

The Patient's Responsibilities on pp. 66–67 reprinted courtesy of Memorial Sloan-Kettering Cancer Center. Copyright © 1999 by Memorial Sloan-Kettering Cancer Center.

A hardcover edition of this book was published in 2000 by HarperCollins Publishers.

First Quill edition published 2001.

Designed by Jackie McKee

The Library of Congress has catalogued the hardcover edition as follows:
Holland, Jimmie C.
     The human side of cancer/Jimmie Holland and Sheldon Lewis—1st ed.
       p. cm.
     Includes index.
     ISBN 0-06-017371-8
     1. Cancer—Psychological aspects. 2. Cancer—Psychosomatic aspects.
     3. Mind and body therapies. I. Lewis, Sheldon. II. Title.
     RC262 .H654 2000
     616.99'4'0019—dc21   00-027583

ISBN 0-06-093042-X (pbk.)

05 ❖/RRD 10 9 8 7 6

For my parents, my husband, and my children—J.H.

For Sheila, Ezra, and Zachary, and for Ed and Denny Levy—S.L.

We are not ourselves when nature, being oppressed,
commands the mind to suffer with the body.

—William Shakespeare, *King Lear*

Poor little old human beings—they're jerked into this world without
having any idea where they came from or what it is they are supposed
to do, or how long they have to do it in. Or where they are
gonna wind up after that. But bless their hearts, most of them
wake up every morning and keep on trying to make some sense
out of it. Why, you can't help but love them, can you? I just
wonder why more of them aren't as crazy as betsy bugs.

—Fannie Flagg, *Welcome to the World, Baby Girl!*

Dr. Holland, I have these three gremlins in my head. One of them
is on one side saying, "Jack, you're going to lick this—don't worry."
Another gremlin is on the other side saying, "Jack, you dope, you know
you aren't going to make it." And in the middle is this third little guy
who has to make sense of both of them and help me to keep
going on with my life day after day. Sometimes, they get
so loud I can't think, but most of the time I keep them locked up,
and when I'm busy they don't bother me.

—Jack Price, a thirty-seven-year-old man
with malignant melanoma

CONTENTS

ACKNOWLEDGMENTS

The Human Side of Cancer is an amalgam of thoughts and knowledge from many people. First and foremost are the many patients and their families who shared their experiences with us. Their willingness to express their deepest—and sometimes darkest—feelings was remarkable. We were humbled to learn how courageous people were in the face of overwhelming problems. The stories in this book are a composite of our experiences in talking with them, with names and circumstances changed to ensure their privacy. A few patients (who became friends) stand out for special mention: Bob Fisher, who started our patient-to-patient counseling program while he was being treated for leukemia. He insisted that our work had to get out to others. His message: "Write the book and forget the science—just tell it from the heart." Others include Jay Weinberg, Jack and Rhonda Price, Karen Swymer, and Sheila Kussner. Also, Cornelia Perry stands tall for her insistence, as a teacher of public speaking, that "you must get the message out about how important this human side of cancer truly is."

Several people who had been through an experience with cancer agreed to read drafts of the book. Gratitude for their work to ensure credibility goes to: Renata Laqueur, Gene Baranoff, and Arlene Eisenberg. Avis Meehan, director of public affairs at Memorial, reviewed the manuscript and made helpful suggestions.

After we have recognized our debt to the patients, the many colleagues who contributed deserve to be mentioned. Those who work with us at Memorial are central: Marguerite Lederberg, with her consistent, quiet, thoughtful advice; Sarah Auchincloss, who taught us about the sexual issues; Mary Jane Massie, who helped start the program at Memorial; Bill Breitbart and Sherry Schacter, who brought the experience of caring for very ill patients at home; Andy Roth; Reverend Tom McDonnell; Jamie Ostroff; Bruce Rapkin; Reverend George Handzo and the Chaplaincy Service; Jesus Almanza; Mindy Greenstein; Alice Kornblith; Donna J. Wilson; our Spiritual Beliefs Seminar group; the Patients to Patients Volunteers; Karrie Zampini; the groups at the Post-Treatment Resource Center at Memorial; and Elizabeth Peabody and the lung cancer support group. All contributed to different aspects of the book. We also thank the psychiatry department staff, especially Ivelisse Belardo.

The work of many researchers and clinicians around the world is cited; these dedicated investigators have contributed, through their studies and insights, to our present knowledge, on which the book is based. We thank Carole Levine and the United Hospital Fund of New York for allowing us to include information from her study on caregivers.

On a personal level, we thank our families who patiently listened and commented on the book. Without Jim Holland, acting as both a supportive spouse and an objective oncologist, the medical underpinnings of the book would have suffered. Encouragement for the book's progress was a part of many conversations with Steven and his wife, Maryland, Mary, Peter and Anne, David, and Diane Holland. Sally Holland and Demece, her partner, read drafts and offered painful but sound criticism.

We are also grateful to Sheila Lewis, who likewise contributed her expertise as an editor and teacher, and to Ezra and Zach. We thank other special friends of this project: Joy Harris, not only a superb literary agent but also a passionate advocate for the human side of cancer, Megan Newman, our editor, for her guidance; Barbara Graham; Ed and Denny Levy; Mark Matousek; Margarita Danielian; and David McMullen.

Finally it was Tony Marchini, our assistant who prepared and organized background materials and provided draft after draft, who made it happen. His unflagging devotion and commitment to the project, his attention to each detail, and his repeated critiques—coupled with confidence in the outcome—ensured its successful completion.

The
HUMAN SIDE
of CANCER

1

WHAT *IS* THE HUMAN SIDE OF CANCER?

I assume that you've picked up this book for the same reasons people come to see me.* You may have just found out you have cancer, or you may already be undergoing treatment and feel you've hit a snag. Perhaps you are a survivor wondering whether you're cured or not. Or you are coping with cancer as a chronic disease and feel the need for more support. Maybe you are a fellow traveler on the path, supporting and assisting a loved one with cancer, but feeling the need for help yourself.

Whatever your situation, I wish I could sit with you and talk about what's been going on for you and how you've been coping, and help you find the kind of support that's right for you. That's the way I would like to do it. But since that's impossible, I've tried through the chapters of this book to talk with you as I would if you were in my office and we were talking face-to-face about your illness or that of your loved one and about the problems you've had to deal with along the way.

When I see someone for the first time at our counseling center at Memorial Sloan-Kettering Cancer Center in New York, I usually ask a question like this: "How have things been going for you since you got sick?"

Often the response is: "I don't even know where to start."

---

*Throughout this book, pronouns in the first person singular refer to Jimmie C. Holland, M.D.

And I usually say: "Well, let's start with your illness. Tell me about what's happened to you."

Then I hear about a "cancer journey," starting with finding a lump or having a pain that took the person to the doctor, who diagnosed cancer. Or, for others, it's how they were completely surprised by the results of a routine mammogram or colonoscopy or chest X ray that showed cancer. Somewhere along the line, each has heard a version of the words "It's cancer."

Some people come to see me at that moment, right after hearing the news, when they are scared, mixed up, and overwhelmed to the point that they can't take the next step. Others come later, after starting their treatment. They hit a "bump in the road" as they cope with radiation or chemotherapy. A psychological "bump" might be feeling "wired" or scared, not being able to sleep or to concentrate on anything, feeling tired and down in the dumps, or being uncertain about the future.

These feelings lead to questions like these: Can I get through this? Is there a light at the end of the tunnel? Will I have done it all for nothing?

Ironically, some people don't come to see me until their treatment is over. They handled treatment fine because they were in a crisis mode and were doing something to fight the cancer. Now that the treatment is completed, they begin to reflect on what they've been through. The reality sets in, and the nagging question arises that I hear so often: *Did* I have cancer, or *do* I have cancer?

Sometimes it's not the person with cancer who comes to see me at all, but a family member or other loved one who finds it painful to watch as the person encounters the curves, valleys, and hills of the cancer journey.

With each of these people, whatever their situation, we talk about how difficult it's been for them to get to where they are now. They often have looked only at their personal shortcomings in meeting the day-to-day crises, seeing only the trees and not the forest. I help them focus on the bigger picture, which so many times reveals how remarkably strong and courageous they have been in the face of one of life's gravest challenges: the threat to life itself.

Together, we look for their inner sources of strength and try to identify their well-honed ways of dealing with adversity that have worked in the past and will likely work again. We review what they know about their cancer and what treatments are out there, and I help them get more information when they need it. We go over their reactions to the diagnosis, their problems with treatment, and their stress as they see family, friends, and coworkers adjusting to the illness of someone close.

Every person brings unique characteristics to dealing with ill-ness: a particular personality, a way of coping, a set of beliefs and val-ues, a way of looking at the world. The goal is to take these qualities into consideration and make sure that they work in favor of the per-son at each point along the cancer journey. I hope that my sugges-tions, impartial information, and sharing of what I have learned over many years of clinical work can make your own journey a little eas-ier and keep you from losing hope.

When I first arrived at Memorial Sloan-Kettering in 1977, very little was known about the human side of cancer. Psychosocial research related to cancer was so new it was hardly viewed as a sci-entific endeavor. But we began to learn about it from the *real* experts: the patients and their families who were going through the experience. Those of us who shared in this exciting beginning at Memorial Sloan-Kettering felt the joy of "discovery"—of being pioneers—as we identified common threads in what we heard, while recognizing that the experience for each individual was unique.

Our work has spanned two decades during which cancer came "out of the closet," allowing the word *cancer* finally to be spoken aloud and the diagnosis honestly given in the United States, as com-pared with many other countries where the diagnosis is still not revealed. Survival from certain cancers has become much more common, and concern for the psychological dimension of patient care has taken on greater importance. Over the past twenty years, we have played a role in the creation of a new subspecialty in cancer (or oncology), which is called *psycho-oncology,* referring to the psycho-logical issues in cancer. Our work at Memorial and the short history of this field are very much intertwined.

During more than twenty years directing the psychiatry effort at

Memorial Sloan-Kettering Cancer Center, I have been listening to patients and their families as they have confronted cancer and struggled to gain a perspective on an unexpected and unwanted intrusion that threatened their own or a loved one's very existence. I have been privileged to witness their remarkable courage and strength. I am grateful for the knowledge and insights that these extraordinary people have shared with me. To have helped some in their journey through the cancer experience has been an even greater privilege that has more than countered the stresses and challenges of the work.

I began to wonder if the knowledge gained from working with well over a thousand patients and their families could be helpful to others facing cancer. Many of my patients have asked, "Can you tell me what to read to help me cope better and get through this?" That's been hard to answer because there are so many books on coping with cancer. I wondered if I dare add one more to the shelves of bookstores. However, many of those books tout a particular approach and promise that it alone will lead to successful coping. If I have learned anything over the years, it is that there is no single right approach and no simple answer to dealing with the human side of cancer.

Although there are some universals about the cancer experience, particularly the sense of uncertainty people feel, we are each as distinct from one another in our psychological dimension as we are in the pattern of our fingerprints and our DNA. It has always seemed unlikely to me, given this diversity, that there is a single right answer for everybody. I tend to doubt any person who says, "I have *the* answer for you."

In addition, cancer has been so frightening for so many years that myths and beliefs have developed that add to the fears. Some of these myths include:

- You wanted to have cancer.

- The problems from your difficult childhood caused it.

- Your negative attitude is making the tumor grow faster.

These beliefs are certainly touted by some who support a particular psychological approach. Many people can put these ideas aside, but others cannot. They are harmful, especially to vulnerable people, who are unable to seek their own independent conclusions. There is no scientific basis for these beliefs, which place an unconscionable added burden on patients who already have enough to cope with. My reason for writing this book is to help you and others "sort out" fact from fiction and belief from reality and to help you along your cancer journey. There is much that we do know from our scientific research and clinical experience that can help you gain a better perspective on your own reactions and emotions. It helps to see your emotions in relation to what others have experienced and to read what the experts in the field have learned.

There are two aspects to the human side of cancer: what cancer does psychologically to people and their families, and how emotions and behaviors may influence the risk of getting cancer and its outcome. In this book we explore both questions, providing practical yet scientifically supported information about the range of issues involved in coping with cancer. We try to help you to find your own best way of coping. We also put into perspective what is known, and what is not known, about the role of the mind and emotions both in getting cancer and in surviving it.

Whenever I read a book, I first want to know something about the author so that I can better judge the book's contents and its reliability. For this reason, I feel you have a right to know "where I'm coming from."

From a personal perspective, the journey to psycho-oncology has been both challenging and rewarding. I always wanted to be a doctor, growing up on a farm during the Depression in what was then called the "blackland Bible-totin'" area of northeast Texas. I greatly admired the country doctor in our little town of Nevada, Texas, who took care of all generations of a family and knew their strengths and foibles. He treated his patients for their range of health problems, from the physical to the psychological. His tools, beyond understanding and empathy, were limited, for treatment of both mind and body. But he made a difference in people's lives, and I wanted to do something like that, though I had never heard of a woman being a doctor. With remarkable support from my parents and several special teachers, I went to medical school.

I loved all of medicine and taking care of patients. But in my internship, I found that listening to people's stories of how they became ill and how they were dealing with their illness was more interesting to me than caring for the physical aspects of their heart trouble or high blood pressure. It was compelling to observe many people with the same illness and similar symptoms and to note the striking differences in their emotional reactions. The reactions ranged from quiet, effective coping in some to a sense of panic and helplessness in others. Making my rounds from room to room, I noticed that some were consumed by fear and sadness—I could hear the fear in their voices and see the terror in their eyes—while others with the same illness seemed optimistic and hopeful about the future. Sometimes people were so upset that they were simply unable to go through the treatments they needed to be cured. I wondered why one person coped so well, while another had such a hard time. What factors led to these very different responses to the same illness? And how could one help those having trouble coping? I became keenly interested then in understanding how people faced the crisis of an illness that threatened their life and the factors that seemed to influence good or poor coping. The pursuit of this interest led me eventually to my work in the field of cancer.

Wanting to understand people's adjustment to illness led me to seek training in psychiatry. Following my residency in psychiatry, in 1956, I met and married a brilliant young oncologist, James Holland. Jim was in the vanguard of doctors who at the time were developing combinations of chemotherapy drugs that drastically changed the outlook for children with acute lymphocytic leukemia from universally fatal to frequently curable. It was an exciting time in cancer medicine as new, effective drugs appeared each year, and the future for cure of cancer looked bright with the prospect of combining surgery, radiation, and chemotherapy. In the early years of our marriage, I mainly stayed at home in Buffalo and took care of our five young children. I would listen to Jim and his colleagues, who often came to dinner, discuss the new treatments for leukemia and the side effects patients had to tolerate to achieve the long-term goal of cure.

Our children began to wonder if there was any world other than that of patients and medicine.

As these pioneer doctors and investigators tried new drugs with patients, they measured and recorded every physical side effect and toxicity the new agents caused. Those long discussions over dinner of the troubling side effects would lead to my asking, "But how do the patients *feel* about all this?" At that time, virtually no one queried the patients about how they were doing because the focus was on changing the dismal outlook all of them faced. Little was known about and little was done to help with the human side of cancer. One patient, Dan, described the situation very well: "They have measured everything but my thoughts and mind. Somehow, my mental attitude, the stress, the anguish should be analyzed and studied the same as my physical condition."

I felt that Dan had put his finger on the problem. If we could measure what our patients were feeling psychologically, we would be able to add that information to the overall assessment of side effects and toxicity. This approach would give us much valuable information, not only about the physical but also about the human effects of a new treatment. That information could then be shared with patients contemplating taking the treatment.

Over the past twenty years, that very thing has happened. I have been privileged to be part of some of the earliest studies that began to seek patients' own reports of their quality of life and level of functioning, not relying only on what the doctors observed. It took a long time for Dan's plaintive observation of the need for measuring his mind and thoughts to be put into practice, but it has happened. And this shift has improved the care of patients by incorporating their concerns and experience, especially as to their pain and distress.

Up until the 1970s, the word *cancer* traditionally was rarely spoken to the patient. Medical schools taught that it was cruel for a doctor to tell patients their diagnosis of cancer (although the family was always informed), since to give the diagnosis would take away all hope, it being tantamount to a death sentence. Since the 1970s, the trend has completely reversed. The decade of the 1970s saw the appearance of women's, patients', and consumers' rights. The post-Vietnam restructuring of American society gave greater attention (and legal sanction) to informing people of their diagnosis and treatment options and to allowing them to make an informed choice of treatment. Today, almost all patients in the United States are told their diagnosis and possible treatments. In some states, legal mandates have been imposed regarding information about particular procedures. For example, some states require that women with early breast cancer be informed of the option to have a lumpectomy and radiation instead of a mastectomy.

Many other countries still cling to the belief that the diagnosis should be withheld from the patient. However, the trend toward openness is becoming more widespread as people the world over become better informed.

Up through the 1950s and 1960s, cancer carried a stigma for the patient and the family, partly owing to the poor survival rate, enforcing a silence on all concerned. Cancer was called the Big C, because the word itself was still so scary. A taxi driver once refused to drive me to Memorial saying, "No ma'am, that place is for the Big C. I drive all the way around it." Many patients felt guilty for bringing the shame of cancer on the family. This cultural silence and stigma limited the opportunity for people even to talk with one other about their illness.

Fanny Rosenow, who became a stalwart volunteer for the American Cancer Society in New York, told me of her experience. In the early 1950s, she and her friend Teresa Lasser had radical mastectomies for breast cancer at the same time. They talked with each other and shared their feelings, but they recognized that most other women had no one with whom to talk about their surgery. Sitting at Fanny's kitchen table, the women decided they would try to reach other women to provide a forum in which women could feel free to talk about having breast cancer. Both women were socially prominent New Yorkers, and Ms. Rosenow felt that a notice in the *New York Times* was the best way to announce such a meeting for women with breast cancer. When she called the *Times*, she was put through to the society editor. Her request to place an ad to announce a meeting about breast cancer for women was followed by a long pause. "I'm sorry, Ms. Rosenow, but the *Times* cannot publish the word *breast* or the word *cancer*. Perhaps you could say there will be a meeting about diseases of the chest wall." Ms. Rosenow hung up in disgust. However, the women persisted, and their devoted efforts resulted in what is widely known as Reach to Recovery, a worldwide support program for women with breast cancer, administered today through the American Cancer Society.

As our five children got older and I returned to work, I felt that cancer provided the ideal setting for me to study people's reactions to illness. Cancer is made up of diseases that occur at all stages of life and in all parts of the world, where attitudes are vastly different. Cancer may be cured, become chronic, or lead to death. To understand how people in these different situations cope could be a basis for helping people cope better with the uncertainty of a life-threatening illness. This interest led me to do research at Roswell Park Cancer Institute in Buffalo and then at Montefiore Hospital in the Bronx, when our family moved to New York.

I came to Memorial Sloan-Kettering in 1977 to begin the first full-time psychiatric service in a cancer research hospital. When I first joined the staff at Memorial, many of the oncologists couldn't understand why they might need someone from psychiatry, because "these people are *really* sick." My colleague, Dr. Mary Jane Massie, a psychiatrist, and I initially shared a small office that had in it a card table and two chairs. But we spent most of our time on the medical floors talking to patients, families, nurses, and social workers and making rounds with the medical teams. The patients were our teachers, sharing their experiences and exploring with us the personal meaning that cancer had in their lives. We learned how to identify those who were distressed, who needed support and help. We began to understand what the common problems were and how to help people deal with them. The human side of cancer began to be more actively addressed in our cancer center.

In this book we talk about the "human effects" of cancer as opposed to the "physical effects" of cancer, which the oncologists and their staff must treat. It is often not recognized that these human effects are part of every encounter with every doctor and every staff member, irrespective of the stage of the illness or the treatments. It is central to all care, yet it is often unceremoniously relegated to the low-priority category of "I don't have time to deal with that today." But individuals and their families confronting cancer grapple with these human issues every day *and want them to be addressed*. Some are psychological, some are social, and some are existential or spiritual.

The succeeding chapters of this book outline these issues. Chapter 2 deals with the myths and beliefs about cancer, and Chapter 3 presents the current state of knowledge about the mind-body connection and cancer.

A diagnosis of cancer raises existential questions like "Why me?" But what immediately comes to mind for most people is "My God, I could die of this," a thought most healthy people have never or rarely entertained, which is the subject of Chapter 4.

Once a diagnosis of cancer has been made, the need to become a partner with your doctor is critical. A positive doctor-patient relationship can make the cancer treatment—and the whole cancer experience—infinitely easier, as discussed in Chapter 5.

Chapter 6, on coping, gives the needed guidelines on effective ways to cope and when to seek help.

The psychological effects of different treatments and how to deal with them are described in Chapter 7. Initial treatment is given with cure as the goal, and the focus is on tolerating the stresses and problems you have to go through to get the cure. This chapter offers help on how to get through your treatment in the best possible way.

Chapter 8 outlines the most common types of cancers and specific psychosocial issues related to each of them.

The good news is that psychological and social support to bolster you and your family is now increasingly available, as described in Chapter 9. Many programs are tailored for the needs of those who are newly diagnosed, are in treatment, are survivors, or are receiving palliative care (treatment to ensure comfort, both physical and psychological, for the patient and family). These programs have repeatedly been shown to improve quality of life. Counseling and psychotherapy are now more widely available, in hospitals and in the community, for those who need individualized psychological help. For severe distress, a psychiatrist might determine whether a medication is needed, in addition to providing counseling, to reduce anxiety, sleeplessness, and depression, which make it difficult to function. The human side, after long neglect, is finally getting the attention it deserves. We call these approaches "medicine that doesn't come in a bottle," and they are discussed in Chapter 9.

Chapter 10 looks at alternative and complementary therapies, which people increasingly are adding to their conventional cancer treatments.

Chapter 11 is concerned with the survivors of cancer, who carry emotional baggage from the experience. It is easier today, in the still relatively new climate of open conversation about cancer, to be a survivor. Cancer survivors want to know how to stay healthy, how to avoid recurrence and the development of a new cancer.

Chapter 12 gives the guidelines for a healthy lifestyle and for proper screening to ensure early detection. As a survivor, you also want to be certain that family members are protected by good health habits and practices.

Unfortunately, not everyone with cancer will survive. Chapters 13 through 16 bear on matters of importance if the cancer progresses. Chapter 13 explains the new phenomenon of seeing cancer as a chronic illness. Today, palliative and terminal care for patients with advanced disease is an aspect of care whose importance is increasingly recognized throughout the country.

The search for meaning in life after cancer is the theme of Chapter 14. We call this search "the last taboo" because of our society's avoidance of talking about ultimate questions like the meaning of life and death.

Chapter 15 discusses the important issues faced by family members and other loved ones who are caring for an ill person.

Finally, Chapter 16 addresses the nature and facets of bereavement and attempts to help answer the question "How do I go on?"

The human side of cancer is all-encompassing; it's about you, your surroundings, and your experience of the illness. It's based on the kind of person you are; the meaning you attach to illness; the specifics of your illness in terms of its stages, symptoms, and treatment; social attitudes; and the availability of support from others. The mix of your particular circumstances influences the human side, along with basic issues such as whether the disease is localized or has spread, whether people are around to help you, your age, and whether or not you have a strong philosophical belief system.

It has been a rewarding personal journey for me to develop a deeper understanding of the challenges people with cancer and their families face and to appreciate how they manage them so well. This book attempts to share with you this collective wisdom.

If you or a loved one has cancer, particularly if you have recently received the diagnosis, your mind is probably filled with questions and feelings that need to be brought into perspective. Questions like "Will I die of this?" "How will I ever get through this?" or "What can I do to improve my chances of cure and survival?" are normal and to be expected. I hope to answer them in this book.

Similarly, many people who have cancer describe a range of emotions—worry, fear, sadness, anger—that may be intense at times. These are all normal and expected responses to a major crisis. Feeling this way doesn't mean that you are mentally ill or lacking in emotional "stamina." Sometimes these feelings become painfully difficult and interfere with your ability to cope with the illness and carry on with your life. It is important that you know of this range of normal reactions as well as the red flags that indicate you might need some help in handling your feelings. Being seriously depressed and anxious are the most common examples. The good news is that most emotional symptoms are treatable. You can face the reality of cancer much better when complicating psychological problems are reduced.

In this age, with its explosion of information, confusing reports about the role of attitudes, emotions, stress, and personality in cancer can place an added burden on you if you have cancer. We want to relieve this burden by providing reliable information about these matters and by helping you find the best sources and types of psychological support. In so doing, we hope to help you manage the human side of cancer.

THE TYRANNY OF
POSITIVE THINKING

*I got really depressed when people said I should think
positive. I thought, "If that's what I have to do to survive, I'm never going to make it."*

—John, a fifty-two-year-old man with melanoma

*People keep telling me to be upbeat. I say, "Screw you.
I'll be however I please in dealing with this cancer. I've
never been upbeat in my life."*

—Michael, a forty-five-year-old schoolteacher with
recently diagnosed sarcoma

Several years ago, Jane,★ a forty-nine-year-old woman with breast
cancer, came to my office at Memorial Sloan-Kettering Cancer
Center in New York City. She had recently completed her treatment, and her doctor had given her a clean bill of health, meaning
the doctors had found no evidence of cancer in her body. Indeed,
the glow of good health had returned to her cheeks.

But as she entered my office, Jane looked agitated. Her body was
tight and tense. As she sat down, I said, "I've heard the good news
from your doctor. I hear you're doing well."

"That's what *he* says," she replied despondently, "but I feel like
I'm losing the battle."

Puzzled, I asked her, "What makes you feel that way?" She
responded, "Well, my sister gave me a book on how to survive

★To protect the privacy of patients, names and identifying characteristics have been
changed, and in some cases composites are used. When first names only are used, they are
fictitious. However, when full names are given, these are the actual names of patients.

cancer, and it says it's critical to keep a positive attitude. I've tried to stay upbeat through the treatments, but now that they're over, I'm more afraid and worried than ever. I'm sad, and I can't feel positive about anything."

I said, "It must have been hard to stay positive all the time over this past year, because I remember how crummy you felt during those first days after each of your six chemotherapy treatments."

"Yes, it's been hard when I've felt so washed out and tired," she said. "And sometimes I've been so scared and frightened, I wondered if I could get through it. Other times, I've been down and sad and angry that this hit me when I had wanted to do so much for my kids. . . ."

"That sounds right on to me," I said. "I can't imagine how you could have been positive all through this last year when you had to slog through so many difficult tests and treatments."

Jane started to relax a little. "You mean it's okay, and I haven't kept my cancer from being killed off by chemotherapy because I couldn't do what that book said?"

"No, you haven't," I said with a smile. "You're not superwoman, you know. You're wonderfully human and normal. Most people experience the same reactions you've had at some time."

"Great!" she said. "Because I was thinking that if any more people tell me to think positive, I'm going to slug them."

Jane was echoing a refrain I often hear from people with cancer: the notion that feeling sad, scared, upset, or angry is unacceptable and that emotions can somehow make your tumor grow. And the sense that if the person is not in control on the emotional plane all the time, the battle against the disease will be lost. Of course, patients like Jane didn't come up with this notion on their own. It's everywhere in our culture: in popular books and tabloids on every newsstand, on talk shows, in TV movies.

For most patients, cancer is the most difficult and frightening experience they have ever encountered. All this hype claiming that if you don't have a positive attitude and that if you get depressed you are making your tumor grow faster invalidates people's natural and understandable reactions to a threat to their lives. That's what I mean by the tyranny of positive thinking. This problem has been brought to me by well-meaning families who say, for example, "You have to help Dad. He's going to die because he isn't positive and he's not trying." On meeting Dad, I see that he clearly is a stoic, a man who copes well in his own quiet way. Maintaining a positive attitude just isn't his style. Insisting that he put on a happy face and cope in a way that would be foreign to him would actually be an added burden; to rob him of a coping mechanism that has worked before seems unfair, even cruel.

Another downside of this tyranny of positive thinking is that Dad may feel guilty for failing his family if his disease should advance and he had been unable to change to a more Pollyanna-like stance.

Another time, I was called by a woman whose husband had died of lung cancer. In her grief, she blamed herself for his death because she had not gotten him to any cancer support groups that could have taught him mind-body techniques, which she believed might have saved him. I tried to reassure her that she had supported him in every way and that these techniques would not likely have carried the day for him in the face of advanced lung cancer.

ATTITUDES ABOUT GETTING CANCER: BLAMING THE VICTIM

The additional negative consequences of these particular beliefs and myths about cancer lead to another phenomenon: blaming the person for getting cancer. Accusing questions, such as "Why did you *need* to get cancer?" or "You must have *wanted* to have cancer" suggest that the patient must have willed it to happen.

Helen, a young woman with cancer, said to me with great sadness, "I feel as if I have been victimized twice: once because I have a brain tumor for which there is no known cause and a second time because I am blamed, that it's my fault. It just isn't fair."

The late Barbara Boggs Sigmund, who was the mayor of Princeton, New Jersey, became furious at the suggestion that she was somehow to blame for her eye cancer (ocular melanoma) and its spread. In a *New York Times* op-ed piece (Figure 1) she expressed her rage at self-help books that presumed that "I had caused my own cancer" out of a "lack of self-love, need to be ill, or the wish to die, and that consequently, it was up to me to cure it." Ms. Sigmund repudiated the theory that "cancer cells are internalized anger gone on a field trip all over our bodies" or that "rah-rah-sis-boom-bah, I can beat the odds if I only learn to love myself enough."

Figure 1. From *The New York Times*, December 30, 1989

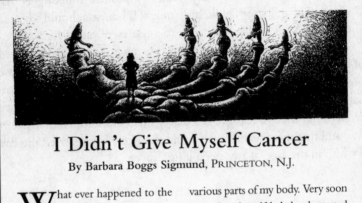

I Didn't Give Myself Cancer

By Barbara Boggs Sigmund, PRINCETON, N.J.

What ever happened to the tragic sense of life?

In late October, a medical exam revealed that my eye cancer—an ocular melanoma—had spread to various parts of my body. Very soon thereafter, the self-help books started arriving. I had caused my own cancer, they told me, so it was up to me to cure it.

I want to set the record straight right up front and give you the most up-to-date information from research studies regarding the role of the mind in causing cancer. It's not your fault that you have cancer. For most cancers, the cause is far from clear, and your psyche did not play a role in your developing it. You surely didn't "want it"! As we learn more about cancer prevention, we are learning about habits and behaviors that do increase cancer risk. But aside from cigarette smoking and lung cancer (see Chapter 12), the results are far from definitive concerning the causes of most cancers.

How did this phenomenon of blaming the patient for the disease come about? It undoubtedly is related to the fact that cancer has been a mystery for so long, as to both cause and cure. When we know little about something, we become even more frightened by it and develop myths to try to explain it and put it in some tolerable perspective. Cancer isn't the first disease to be saddled with myths. Until a cure for tuberculosis using antibiotics was found in the 1940s, it was said that people with certain personality traits developed tuberculosis and that stress or an emotional weakness led to contracting it. Such ideas disappeared as science established that tuberculosis was caused by a bacterial infection and drugs became available to cure it.

I saw some of the first patients with AIDS in New York in the early 1980s. In those early years, fears among the public were high because we didn't know the cause and we didn't know how the disease was transmitted. Many people were terrified until the virus was identified and the blood supply for transfusions was made safe. Panic diminished when scientists identified the highest risk to be from exposure to bodily fluids containing the AIDS virus, through either contaminated needles or sexual contact.

Similarly, as we know more about the causes of cancer and as more types of cancer become curable, the myths surrounding it become less powerful. Increasingly, we depend more on valid scientific information and less on long-held beliefs.

When misfortune strikes, it is a natural human tendency to search for a reason. The ready explanation is often "he must have brought it on himself." This reaction is similar to the response when someone is mugged. People say, "What were you doing in that neighborhood, at night, anyway?" Blaming the victim lets us say, "It can't happen to *me*." This response is a part of a bigger psychological picture: the need to attribute a cause to any catastrophic event, whether an earthquake or an illness. By blaming the victim, we get a false sense of security that we can prevent events that are beyond our control. We seek to make sense of something that surely makes no sense at all.

The fact is we can't always prevent cancer. Susan Sontag makes the strong point in *Illness as Metaphor:*

Illness is the night side of life, a more onerous citizenship.
Everyone who is born holds dual citizenship, in the kingdom
of the well and in the kingdom of the sick. Although we all
prefer to use the good passport, sooner or later each of us is
obliged, at least for a spell, to identify ourselves as citizens of
that other place.

So it makes no sense to blame the person who is ill. Being ill makes one feel alone enough, and being blamed adds to a feeling of distance and isolation, of somehow being "different" from others in a way we've never experienced before. As Robert, a young man with Hodgkin's disease, put it, "I'm not Robert anymore. Now I'm Robert with cancer. I feel alone with it." You may have encountered the blaming response from friends and family members. If so, I advise you to tell them, "I know you have my best interests at heart. But it's not helpful to tell me that I had something to do with my getting cancer. And it's not realistic to expect me to be positive twenty-four hours a day."

ATTITUDES AND SURVIVING CANCER

The same attitudes that are at work in blaming you for having caused the cancer in the first place are often also applied in explaining why you are cured or not. Attitudes and personality, by affecting your behavior, do often lead to your getting an early diagnosis of cancer. This alone is a key factor in cure. For example, if you are the type of person who has a proper respect for staying healthy, you go to the doctor for regular checkups or when troubling symptoms develop, you cooperate with your doctor and follow advice carefully, and by so doing you are apt to discover a cancer at an early stage, should it develop. We know a lot about the ways that our personality and emotions lead us to engage in habits or behaviors that increase our risk of getting cancer. Good examples are smoking and lung cancer, and sunburn and malignant melanoma.

We also know a lot about how attitudes and emotions can affect our endocrine and immune systems as we respond to stress. However, it is less clear whether attitudes and emotions, by themselves, can change an internal process to make an impact on tumor growth or the body's response to it. We don't know whether the blips in hormone and immune levels due to stress have any connection to cancer at all or, should there be any such connection, how it works.

Indeed, research in the new field of *psychoneuroimmunology*— exploring connections between the brain, the hormonal (endocrine) system, and the immune system—has given us an exciting picture of the body's responses to stress. It is known that different types of stress, ranging from taking medical school exams to going through a divorce, affect both hormones and the immune system. The evidence linking stress and risk of heart disease is quite strong. Stress exerts its effect through the nervous system, which in turn affects heart rate, blood pressure, and hormones. But whether this is so for cancer is far less clear. Nevertheless, people today have many questions, based on what they've read and what their friends tell them about cancer and the mind. And people make a lot of mistakes and premature assumptions on the basis of incomplete research. They think, for instance, that if the stress of divorce affects immune function, then it follows that "my divorce must have caused my cancer." This kind of extrapolation, which is without scientific evidence, leads to many false assumptions and conclusions. In Chapter 3, we attempt to separate facts as we know them now from the hype and plain misinformation surrounding the mind-body-cancer connection.

It is common for people who have survived cancer to look back on the experience and attribute their survival to their positive thinking, discounting the fact that they also sought medical help early and had the best-known treatment for their cancer. This belief not only provides an explanation for their cure from cancer, but also buffers fears that it will come back. "If I licked it once with this attitude, then I can keep it from coming back the same way." This belief is reassuring and provides a way of coping with the normal fears people have about the cancer returning. A good attitude surely leads to the best and most logical approach to getting cancer successfully treated. But I have also known people with positive attitudes, who sought early diagnosis and treatment, and who simply weren't as fortunate. I have seen patients who had no belief in the mind-body connection and who discounted the importance of their attitude completely, yet they survived.

> Ernie, a lawyer who was absolutely negative about every aspect of his diagnosis and treatment of lymphoma, was convinced from Day 1 that he would not survive. He explained that he usually saw the dark side of things and the glass as half-empty. Although he stuck faithfully to his chemotherapy treatment, no amount of encouragement or "good" results on his medical tests could persuade him he was doing well. He would say over and over again, "Dr. Holland, I'm not going to make it." It's now been eighteen years since his treatment; he's been cancer free ever since. He's still going strong and is still as much a pessimist as ever. Ernie is an example of how attitude is not the whole story in surviving cancer.

My view is that if a positive attitude comes naturally to you, fine. Some people are optimistic, confident, and outgoing in virtually every situation. Your attitude toward illness reflects your attitude toward life in general and your handling of day-to-day stresses and hassles. There is no way you will see that the glass is half-empty if you are certain that it is half-full. And the converse is true: If you see the glass as half-empty, I can't convince you that it is half-full. It is not easy to change people's ingrained attitudes and patterns of coping.

It's dangerous to generalize about attitudes and their impact on cancer without more information. The present-day tyranny of positive thinking sometimes victimizes people. If thinking positively works for you, well and good. If it doesn't, use the coping style that's natural to you and has worked in the past. (I discuss different modes of coping in Chapter 6.) Trying to get you to "put on a happy face," to pretend you are feeling confident when in fact you are feeling tremendously fearful and upset, can have a downside. By feigning confidence and ease about your illness and its treatment, you may cut off help and support from others. You may also be hiding anxious and depressed feelings that could be alleviated if you told your doctor how you really feel. Also, this tyranny of positive thinking can inhibit you from getting the help you may need out of fear of disappointing your loved ones or admitting to a personality some people think is fatal. If you are surrounded by "the positive attitude police," ask your doctor, clergy, or therapist to call them off, letting them know that this is an important time for you to be honest about your feelings so that you can get all the help you need. (Or give your family or friends this chapter to read.)

It is ironic that many negative, pessimistic people survive cancer, while others who believe positive attitudes will cure it do not. While members of the former group are stunned by their survival, those in the latter group are made to feel guilty or ashamed that they were not "up to" beating an aggressive disease. This is unfair. I do not believe for an instant that people whose cancer progresses have a weaker spirit or character than anyone else.

For many years, whenever I spoke to groups of patients and their families about cancer and the mind, I would cite all the research data suggesting that we couldn't attribute cancer survival totally to personality or positive attitudes. Invariably, someone would come up to me after the talk and say, "Dr. Holland, I heard what you said about the research, and I respect your opinion. But, I don't care about what the research says. I believe in the mind-body connection, and I know I survived because of my attitude." I began to realize that people have strong ideas about these issues that aren't based as much on facts as on deeply held beliefs.

I have come to view beliefs about the mind-body-cancer connection as being similar to beliefs about religion. People who truly believe don't need (or look for) scientific proof of the connection. People who don't believe are equally adamant on the "no connection" side. I have learned from experience that trying to influence strongly held beliefs is exhausting and, more important, successful only once in a blue moon. You believe or you don't. What probably matters most in the long run is that your view is consoling and comforting to you. We have a strong obligation to insist that families and medical staff respect each person's beliefs about cancer. People who have cancer should be supported, irrespective of their views, and without fear of criticism or ridicule from those around them.

Clearly, there is a broad spectrum of beliefs regarding the role of the mind and emotions in cancer. Some people believe that emotions are the key factor and that cancer is caused—and, therefore, can be controlled—by the proper emotional makeup and response. Others discard that idea as unscientific and untenable by current scientific standards. Others sit in the middle, believing that how we respond to cancer certainly affects the quality of our lives—and *might* have an impact on survival.

If you do hold a belief in a mind-body-cancer connection, it is important that you understand that your doctor may not share your view. However, most doctors today are willing to disagree respectfully and do not discourage complementary mind-body therapies that are potentially helpful and not harmful. (A complementary therapy is used in addition to, rather than instead of, standard medical treatment; see Chapter 10.) Most physicians today will say something like this: "I'm not aware of the proof for that. But I encourage you to do anything and everything that helps you feel better, so long as it doesn't interfere with your medical treatment."

Occasionally, a physician might completely discourage you from pursuing a therapy you believe is helping you. It is important to resolve the conflict with your doctor as best you can through open discussion. Even if your doctor does not agree with the approach you've embraced, it is important to be honest about it. For example, if a diet or nutritional regimen you've embarked on has caused you to lose a lot of weight, tell your doctor, because it could interfere with your medical treatment. Most diets suggested today are not extreme, but any that limit protein and calories can reduce your body's ability to tolerate chemotherapy.

Researchers in Toronto, Drs. Brian Doan and Ross Gray, suggest that at one extreme of a continuum of beliefs about the mind and cancer are the persons who see cancer as the enemy and see themselves as the warrior on the white horse who must fight the proverbial dragon, in this case, cancer, like St. George. These are the folks who confidently say, "I'm going to beat this." British researchers Drs. Steven Greer and Maggie Watson, at the Royal Marsden Cancer Institute, called this the "fighting spirit," which ensures that a person uses a head-on, direct approach to dealing with cancer. We know that this is a good way to cope. This active stance is carried a step further in a complementary cancer therapy in which one visualizes the immune system fighting cancer. This approach was developed by Dr. O. Carl Simonton and Stephanie Simonton and popularized in their book *Getting Well Again*.

The Simonton approach encourages patients to visualize their healthy cells fighting the cancer cells. This method is appropriate and satisfying for many people with the fighting spirit. Patients with this personality type derive considerable comfort from visual imagery, relaxation exercises, and hypnosis. These are also people who confront their problems head-on when well, and they are likely to collaborate vigorously in their treatments when ill.

However, this approach is not for everyone. Many people tend to face a difficult situation by using an outwardly "nonfighting," stoic stance. They may view the role of the mind as less central in the treatment of cancer, except as it involves commitment to the medical treatment. In the past several years, these individuals have often been made to feel that they are failing because they cannot create a warriorlike fighting stance. They may be criticized by relatives for "not trying hard enough." Many people with cancer come to see me or other therapists for help with depressed feelings precisely because they don't fit today's popular model for coping with cancer. They assume that it must be their fault that they're out of step, that there must be something wrong with them. So they come to see me in the hope of getting fixed up and altered into a "healthy, normal" coper. Instead, they're often surprised to discover that I validate their feelings and their own natural way of coping. I learned early on that when a person is in the middle of a crisis related to illness, it is not the time to try to change his or her way of coping. When you are in the "trenches" of cancer treatment, it is best for you to call on the resources you already have. Immediate support is important in the crisis. Helping you find more appropriate and more effective ways to cope can come later (see Chapter 6).

If you wake up every morning and exclaim, "I'm going to beat this thing!" and you practice your imagery exercises, which help you feel powerful in the face of this tough disease, I would never discourage you from following this "combat-style" approach to your cancer.

But if you wake up and say, "Oh God, I don't know how I will get through this. I just feel so lousy and scared," you likely need some help to cope better. Nevertheless, as of today's knowledge, you are *not* making your cancer worse.

The bottom line is that there is no generic "one size fits all" coping style for dealing with cancer. If there is one thing we hope to accomplish in this book, it is to make it clear that you are unique, and your tried and true ways of coping (that have worked in past crises) are likely your best bet for dealing with the crises of cancer. I urge family members, friends, and medical professionals to respect and support each person's way of coping.

If you are a "nonbeliever" in the mind-body connection and cancer, it may reassure you to know that the scientific base is not firmly established for such a connection in cancer beyond the important role the mind plays in getting us to the proper medical treatment and maintaining a healthy lifestyle. We really don't know whether psychological or emotional factors play a role in extending life by some as yet not understood mechanism, but the factor is likely to be small in relation to the total picture.

We do have overwhelming proof, however, that how you cope with your illness can improve your overall quality of life. This will clearly lead you to get the best medical results because of a better working relationship with your doctors and your willingness to complete your full course of treatment, which in turn leads to a better outcome from your treatment.

Taking a middle position on this mind-body-cancer subject has not been easy because of the way the "believers" and "nonbelievers" feel so strongly one way or the other. Over the years, some of my colleagues in cancer medicine have viewed me as an advocate of "soft science" regarding mind-body-cancer interactions. At the same time, proponents of mind-body techniques have considered me to be a conservative spokesperson for the medical establishment, lacking the ability to accept their premises without proof.

In all honesty, I am entirely comfortable with my place in the middle of the road, holding an open mind. On the one hand, I firmly believe in the value of scientific research. I would never tell you that a particular technique has been proved effective when, to my mind, the data to support it are not yet there. On the other hand, I encourage you to pursue approaches, proved or not, that help you to feel better, as long as the approach is not harmful and as long as you continue the medical treatment recommended by your physician. Complementary approaches are popular today, and they permit you to feel more in control by personally contributing to the treatment.

You need to find your own comfort level with the mind-body-cancer connection, based on your temperament, your natural way of coping, and your belief system. That approach should be respected by your family, your doctor, and others who support you through the cancer experience.

3

THE MIND-BODY CONNECTION AND CANCER

Did a Life of Tragedy Cause Her Fatal Cancer?
>—Tabloid headline on the death of
>Jacqueline Kennedy Onassis

*I know why I got cancer. It happened right after I lost
my job.*
>—Terence, a forty-year-old man with colon cancer

*If my husband, Ron, hadn't left me, my cancer would
never have come back.*
>—Julia, a forty-nine-year-old woman
>with ovarian cancer

*My terrible childhood with my mother must have
caused my breast cancer.*
>—Jean, a forty-two-year-old woman

*P*eople ask me the same questions with amazing frequency:

Did my personality or emotions cause my cancer?

Did the stress I was under alter my immune system
and cause my cancer?

Did grief or a loss cause my cancer, and could it
make the cancer come back?

When I get down and depressed, am I making my
   tumor grow faster?

How important is support from others?

How can I help make my treatment work?

You may have asked yourself the same questions as well. Here are
my answers based on what we know and don't know.

DID MY PERSONALITY OR EMOTIONS
CAUSE MY CANCER?

Do certain personality traits, a history of adverse childhood experiences, or a particular way of coping with stress make a person more
likely to get cancer and to die from it? Conversely, do other personality or coping patterns protect people from getting cancer or help
them survive it? We know that personality affects lifestyle and habits,
which may lower or raise your cancer risk. If you ignore warnings
about smoking, for example, or continue to engage in other risky
health behaviors, you increase your risk of cancer. Another high-risk
trait is procrastination in seeing a doctor when you have a symptom,
like a persistent cough or rectal bleeding. I call this the "ostrich"
syndrome, which is trying to avoid a problem or deny that it may
exist, out of fear.

One theory suggests that people with repressive personalities, who
look calm but hold in a cauldron of painful emotions, are more prone
to develop cancer. Dr. Lydia Temoshok, a psychologist who led a
number of research studies on personality and cancer at the University
of California, San Francisco, labeled this the Type C personality (by
the way, C doesn't stand for cancer). You are likely to be familiar with
the Type A (hostile, impatient) personality and the Type B (docile, passive) personality, which lead to greater or lesser risk of heart attack.
Type C individuals are in between: They have a dramatic physical
response to stress, yet they report that they are not highly stressed at all.

Although Temoshok and her colleagues found some differences in cancer risk and survival among Type C patients with melanoma, the general consensus in the scientific community is that there is insufficient evidence to make the leap that if you are a Type C, you are more prone to cancer or less likely to survive it than other people.

Another theory suggests that people with a "fighting spirit," who face cancer as a challenge, as if armed for battle, have a better chance of surviving cancer than people who are stoic or passive. To test this theory, Drs. Steven Greer and Maggie Watson at Royal Marsden hospital in London gave women with breast cancer a questionnaire to determine their personality type. Ten years later, they found that women who demonstrated a "fighting spirit" survived longer than women who were stoic or passive. We know today that the primary predictor of survival for women with breast cancer is whether the cancer has spread to the lymph nodes under the arm. But at the time of their research, scientists did not know this, so no one checked the lymph nodes to look for cancer spread. Consequently, this critical predictor was not taken into account in the Greer-Watson study. A more recent study by Dr. Maggie Watson, controlled for medical factors, has found that a "fighting spirit" is not a predictor for survival. The bottom line: Current knowledge tells us that the strongest factor in survival from breast cancer is the presence or absence of positive nodes for cancer, not the personality of the individual. A "fighting spirit" is surely a helpful way to cope, but we don't know that it directly influences survival.

Over the years, many studies have been conducted to clarify the role of personality in health. The studies have frequently found contradictory or inconclusive results. This is largely because of the difficulty in carefully studying psychological and physical domains at the same time. It is natural, therefore, for people to throw up their hands and say, "They really don't know what they're doing" or "How can they get such conflicting results—they can't all be right!" But scientists tolerate these differences, recognizing that it takes many studies to gather sufficient information to prove a fact with certainty.

In conducting research, we struggle with the question: Did we control all the factors so that no "red herring" could account for the results? This is the only way we can be sure that our results are accurate. The best studies today try to avoid these glitches by carefully considering and "controlling" all relevant factors.

Rather than trying to pin cancer risk on certain personality types, research in recent years has explored the role of our coping patterns: How we handle daily hassles in our life relates to how we deal with cancer and its outcome. Certainly, if your personality leads you to go to a doctor quickly with a symptom that might be cancer, you likely get an earlier diagnosis, which will more probably lead to cure. If you procrastinate, cancer may be diagnosed later, at a less curable stage. Other personality traits, such as tenacity and persistence, play a role in determining whether you doggedly hang in to complete the treatment.

The myth of the cancer personality is akin to the tyranny of positive thinking (discussed in the previous chapter). Jesse, a fifty-one-year-old college professor with Hodgkin's disease, summed up the controversy this way:

> *What difference does it make telling me my personality might have given me cancer? It's like telling me my blue eyes caused cancer. Even if it were true, I can't change it. Tell me something I can do something about.*

Jesse's right. You can't change the enduring parts of your personality. However, you *can* use your ways of coping to advantage by maintaining a healthy lifestyle, seeking care if you have a symptom suggestive of cancer or one that is unexplained for weeks, and hanging in with the treatment if it is cancer.

DID STRESS ALTER MY IMMUNE SYSTEM AND CAUSE MY CANCER?

Many research studies have shown that stressful life events, from the death of a loved one to the loss of a job, are linked to an increase in certain health problems, particularly heart disease, diabetes, and hypertension. Many people assume that stress must lead to cancer as well. Evidence for this, however, is not clear. For the time being, there is no proof that the hormonal and mild immune system blips caused by stress influence the onset or progression of cancer.

What we know about stress is that when we are confronted with a frightening situation, we mobilize our brain and our body to deal with it. The acute (immediate) stress response turns on the autonomic (self-regulating) nervous system, which controls basic functions like breathing and heart rate; they go on without your thinking about them. Dr. Walter Cannon in the 1920s first described the "fight-or-flight response." Later, Dr. Hans Selye, the pioneer researcher in stress, termed it the "emergency response," when he explored the effect on the endocrine (hormonal) and immune systems. The body marshals its hormones and immune system to fight whatever is attacking it, either externally or internally. Parts of the immune system (the white blood cells) are "traffic cops," whose job is to ward off infection. These cells race to a cut on your arm or an infection in your throat. This positive and critically important part of the stress response gears up the human body for meeting a challenge inside the body.

Studies by Drs. Ronald Glaser and Janice Kiecolt-Glaser of Ohio State University have shown that many different types of stress trigger changes in the immune system. Medical students taking examinations have short-term changes, while people caring for a relative with Alzheimer's disease have long-term, continuous stress and more prolonged changes in immune function. How do these clearly proven facts relate to cancer? Breast cancer surgery alone causes slight temporary changes in the immune system, but women with higher levels of distress who had the surgery showed a greater change in some parts of immune function, according to a study by Dr. Barbara Anderson, a psychologist at Ohio State University. Put simply, there's an immune system blip from surgery alone, but the blip is greater if you are distressed. It is a big leap, though, to go from this finding to saying that stress affects the outcome of breast cancer. The bottom line is that the mind-body connection is clear—emotions affect hormones and immune function—but that the link between mind-body interactions and cancer is far less clear and remains unproved. There is a vast differ-ence between saying that stress temporarily alters some functions of the immune system and saying that stress, therefore, causes cancer.

Dr. Bruce McEwen, a brain researcher at Rockefeller University in New York City, carried this research forward. In an article in the *New England Journal of Medicine* in 1998, he described a theory of how chronic stress causes "wear and tear" on the body. Stress affects all of us every day, ranging from minor to major events; we react and return to normal. McEwen calls this phenomenon *allostasis.* He suggested, how-ever, that the physiological changes associated with stress over long periods result in an "allostatic load," which, simply put, is the wear and tear that makes us more vulnerable to heart disease, non-insulin-dependent diabetes, hypertension, and infections such as the common cold. McEwen's contribution to this intriguing area is important. He suggests that we can offset this wear and tear and minimize the allo-static load by keeping the body in shape with exercise and nutrition, and by keeping our stress at a tolerable level. If you cope with crisis by assessing it objectively and staying calm, you likely reduce the body's stress. If you deal with crises that way and rarely panic, you likely have a lower allostatic load, as described by McEwen.

In relation to cancer, however, stress-related changes in the endocrine and immune systems have not, so far, been persuasively linked to increased risk or survival. Studies that have taken into account the known predictors, such as extent of tumor spread and type of treatment, have not found stress to be a major factor.

DID GRIEF OR A LOSS CAUSE MY CANCER, AND COULD IT MAKE THE CANCER COME BACK?

One of the most strongly held beliefs in our society is that depres-sion, grief, or loss of a loved one can lead someone to "die of a broken heart." Literary accounts of such consequences abound, depicting the surviving partner not wanting to live on alone. When a grieving spouse develops cancer, it is assumed that the cancer occurred as a response to the loss.

Grief has come under study in recent years, both the psychological and physical aspects. (Chapter 16 is devoted to this topic.) An expert panel was convened several years ago by the Institute of Medicine to look at what is known about grief and its psychological and physical consequences. This panel of experts reviewed all available studies and confirmed the well-known profound feelings of sadness and loss. But when the reviewers looked at the available studies to determine whether grief increased a person's vulnerability to disease and death, and particularly death from cancer, the overall evidence was far less compelling.

I remember June, who came to see me because she was fearful that the recent death of her husband might cause her breast cancer to recur. Several studies suggest that this is not true, despite findings that grief does transiently affect the immune system. Twenty years ago, research conducted at Mount Sinai Medical Center in New York and in Australia involved men in the nine months following their wives' death from breast cancer. The study found that the men had negative changes in some cells of their immune system for a period of several months.

This result led to concern about whether the immune changes would raise the risk for developing cancer in these men and among grieving individuals in general. Several studies have been conducted to determine whether there is greater mortality from cancer among people who have had a loss. Researchers from Israel, Denmark, and the United States have examined the impact of losing a spouse or a child, since these are the most significant losses people experience. Ten years after the loss, the surviving spouses and parents had no greater mortality from cancer than those who did not experience a loss during that period.

The studies in Israel and Denmark were of parents who had lost a child. In Israel, the parents had lost sons in battle during the Six-Day War or in an accident; in Denmark, the parents had lost children to leukemia. Death rates for these bereaved parents were no greater overall than among those who had not suffered such a loss. Cancer did not appear more frequently as a cause of death than would normally be expected, suggesting strongly that grief does not increase the risk of getting cancer, despite the enormity of the loss.

These epidemiological data strongly suggest that the transient immune changes found by the Mount Sinai group and others in bereaved individuals are not sufficient to increase the risk of developing cancer. As intuitive as it feels that grief may make a person vulnerable to cancer, there are as yet no data supporting the notion.

What if you already have cancer? Will a loss cause the cancer to come back or progress? In a study done through a cancer clinical trials group, my colleagues and I investigated whether the loss of a spouse or child would cause women who had been treated for breast cancer to have a recurrence sooner or to have a shorter survival time. We conducted a study of several hundred women who had received the same adjuvant chemotherapy for Stage II breast cancer. We compared the women who had lost a child or spouse since receiving chemotherapy treatment with women who had no loss during the same seven years. Unlike some studies reporting that a loss led to a recurrence of breast cancer, here the two groups of women were matched on important medical factors known to predict survival (like number of positive nodes under the arm and estrogen receptor status). There was no difference in recurrence or in survival. This is reassuring information for women who have had breast cancer and fear that the loss of someone dear will cause their cancer to begin to grow. You can reassure others of the fact that sustaining a loss doesn't bring on a return of cancer. Several other studies have shown similar results.

Evelyn is a good example of someone who feared that loss could set the stage for the return of her cancer.

A young teacher of thirty-five with two small children, Evelyn had been treated for Stage II breast cancer by lumpectomy and radiation, followed by chemotherapy. Her life was getting back on track when her mother, age seventy, developed a recurrence of a breast cancer that had occurred five years earlier. Her mother died. Evelyn had been close to her mother and grieved deeply for her. She and her husband came to see me in panic out of concern that Evelyn's breast cancer might return because of her grieving so painfully for her mother. We worked on helping her express her sense of loss and the understandable fears it generated in her. I reassured her that careful research studies did not support her strong belief that grieving would cause her breast cancer to return. After four months, she felt more like her usual self, relieved that her grieving was normal and necessary and that sadness would not cause her cancer to return.

WHEN I GET DOWN AND DEPRESSED, AM I MAKING MY TUMOR GROW FASTER?

Patrick, a marketing representative with melanoma, asked whether depression, either mild or "full-blown," leads to cancer. The answer, according to most reliable scientific studies, is no. A large study in which people were randomly chosen in several representative cities looked at depressed individuals ten years after they were identified as having either clinical depression or milder symptoms. There was no increased mortality from cancer among them, compared with those who had not experienced depression. This fact, however, is in sharp contrast to the results of research concerning depression and heart disease.

The bottom line, as far as we can say now, is that neither grief, depression, nor depressed feelings increase a person's risk of developing cancer or of progression of a cancer.

HOW IMPORTANT IS SUPPORT FROM OTHERS?

An intriguing and increasingly important aspect of health is our sense of connection to other people, both at a personal level (with friends and relatives, for example) and at the level of feeling part of a community. At first glance, this subject might appear to have little relation to disease vulnerability or survival, but it actually is emerging as an important factor.

First, it is clear that ties to others affect our health. Many studies have found that both men and women who have more social connections have a lower death rate from all causes than is expected for persons their age. But those who are isolated, with little connection to others, have the highest mortality from all diseases. Drs. Peggy Reynolds and George Kaplan, at the University of Michigan, found in a large study that having more social ties was associated with lower mortality, including mortality from cancer, but that being married did not have this effect. Marriage can be a plus or a minus, as today's divorce rate confirms.

A study of specific aspects of social ties found that involvement in a range of social activities, as well as the quality of relationships and frequency of contacts (not necessarily the numbers of friends or acquaintances), were the most important elements.

How could social support versus isolation affect your health? The first and obvious explanation is that when you have someone who cares about you, you are more likely to get to the doctor when you need to, pay more attention to good diet, and avoid less healthy habits. It may be as simple as that. However, there is little doubt that, when you have someone with whom you can share the burden of your illness, it becomes less threatening and you feel a greater sense of control and confidence than if you were alone. More social support and contacts may lower your distress, therefore, and help you cope better with your illness. While we don't know how social ties are translated into an effect on survival, the evidence that they are seems clear and compelling enough to make researchers want to study them more.

It's important to keep in mind that if you tend to have few social connections and function well that way, it's likely a long-held pattern that has worked for you and one to which your body has adapted over many years. Still, if you're comfortable socializing or can overcome shyness, my "prescription" would be to try to develop ties to a few people. Volunteering for a charity or belonging to a club, organization, or religious group fulfills this need for many people. Friendships grow out of these contacts.

The bottom line is this: Positive involvement with others appears important in helping you to maintain good health habits and live longer.

CAN SUPPORT GROUPS HELP ME LIVE LONGER?

A question I heard from a young man, John, facing testicular cancer, was: "Can joining a support group help improve my chances?" Groups have become popular as a means of support among patients. They got an enormous boost in 1989 when Dr. David Spiegel, a psychiatrist at Stanford University, reported a ten-year study showing that women receiving standard treatment for metastatic breast cancer who had participated in group therapy lived longer by an average of eighteen months. The study was not originally designed to look at survival, and the women were never told that group sessions might influence their survival. Published in the British medical journal *Lancet*, this study created a great stir in the medical community and among patients. People with cancer began to seek out groups more actively, and some professionals suggested that support groups be included (and covered by insurance) as part of standard cancer treatment. The study turned out to be a great stimulus for the popularization of group support for patients and for research into group therapies.

These were results that everybody wanted to hear: patients, families, mental health workers, and oncologists. If group therapy could not only improve quality of life but help people to live longer, there could not be better news. The study awaits replication by Spiegel and others to confirm that groups can affect both quality of life and survival. Some subsequent studies have not found an increase in survival. Since it is difficult to control all factors, questions have been raised as to whether some factor not considered in the study might have influenced the positive result found by Spiegel.

A second study, by Drs. Fawzy, a husband–and–wife research team at UCLA, found that patients with malignant melanoma benefited psychologically from group sessions following surgery, focused on giving patients information about their disease and providing emotional support for them. Five years later, of the thirty-five patients studied, those who participated in the group shortly after their diagnosis were disease-free longer and survived longer overall. The longer-term survival (ten years or more) has not been reported.

Research is needed to confirm these findings, particularly since so few patients were studied.

In two other studies, patients participating in support groups did not live longer. Dr. Bernie Siegel, who started the Exceptional Cancer Patient (ECaP) program, and investigators at the Bristol Clinic in England found similar negative results.

However, as I discuss in Chapter 9, the groups available today, such as the Wellness Community and Gilda's Clubs, do a tremendous job of improving life for patients. I strongly support patients' joining groups, if they personally find them helpful. When my patients ask me if they should join a support group, I say that we know that groups can improve quality of life and decrease distress for many patients, but the jury is still out regarding their effect on lengthening life.

HOW CAN I HELP TO MAKE MY TREATMENTS WORK?

How can you use this information about the mind-body connection in your own care? First, you must be wondering what you can really believe. This is understandable; we mentioned earlier that there are believers and nonbelievers in the mind-body connection. People vary in how much store they place in *any* psychological research. Nonbelievers consider such research "touchy-feely"; believers care less about data because they feel certain that the connection exists. What we have tried to present here is a balanced view of this most controversial aspect concerning psychological issues in cancer.

My best advice to you for now is to take a rational and reasoned approach. Take news reports with a wait-and-see, grain-of-salt attitude. Don't rush to change your general approach to coping with cancer. Good attitudes and good access to support, including groups, can help.

Here are some conclusions you can reasonably draw from the facts put forward in this chapter:

1. You can help yourself most by adopting healthy habits and healthy lifestyle (see Chapter 12).

2. See a doctor if you have any symptom that is suggestive of cancer or if you have an unexplained symptom that persists. Early diagnosis ensures the best outcome.

3. Don't blame yourself. You can't cause cancer by having a particular personality.

4. Stick with the medical treatment your doctor recommends. It's your best shot for survival.

5. Your coping style is personal and unique. There is no single right way to cope. Use what works for you.

6. If your way of coping isn't working, ask for professional help.

7. Stress, depression, and grief do not increase the likelihood that cancer will develop or that it will come back if you've been treated before.

8. Although stress causes blips in hormone and immune functions, they have not been linked to increased risk of cancer or poorer survival.

9. Support groups help reduce distress and the feeling of loneliness. Some studies suggest that they may affect survival, although we don't have proof for that. If you aren't a "grouper," and don't find groups helpful, don't feel you are adversely affecting your health by not joining one.

These issues are discussed in more detail in Chapter 6, where you will find a list of Do's and Don't's for coping.

4

THE DIAGNOSIS:
"I COULD DIE OF THIS"

My doctor was very matter-of-fact. He said, "The tumor is malignant. We can do such and such treatments, and this and this will happen." But I could barely hear a word he said. The whole time I was thinking, "My God, I have cancer! I could die!"

—Maria, a fifty-four-year-old woman
with ovarian cancer

The first chapter should be "Am I Gonna Die?" because that's what everyone thinks about when they're first diagnosed.

—Children with cancer to Erma Bombeck for her
book *I Want to Grow Up, I Want to Grow Hair,
I Want to Go to Boise: Children Surviving Cancer*

THE WORKUP

Many people's first experience with cancer begins quite simply with the discovery of a symptom or sign known to be a possible cancer indicator. A breast lump, a sore that has changed in appearance or hasn't healed properly, any persistent severe pain, blood in the stool or urine, a sore throat or cough that persists—these are several of the most common signs. From this moment, the uncertainty of cancer begins. Could this symptom mean cancer, or can I assume it's nothing?

But this moment, before the doctor has even been called or a single test has been done, often transforms a person's life from one of general well-being and confidence to one of enormous anxiety and uncertainty about the future. This pervasive sense of uncertainty probably characterizes the journey with cancer more than anything else. It often lessens when things are going well, but it is a feeling that never completely goes away. This seems to be what people mean when they say, "The diagnosis completely changed my life." That wonderful sense of certainty and expectation of continued life and health, a kind of denial that the bubble can ever burst, is destroyed. Learning to live with uncertainty becomes the bottom line in dealing with cancer.

Many people who notice a "suspicious" symptom have encountered cancer before through the illness of a loved one, such as a parent or grandparent. If a symptom suggests that you might have the same type of cancer as your loved one had, you may become terrified. Fear that you might go through the same vividly recalled cancer experience as someone close to you did can be overwhelming. In such cases, a person may be too frightened to go to a doctor. A sense of hopelessness—if it's cancer, nothing can be done—or a feeling of panic can paralyze your ability to act. This was the case for a man, Brett, who told me that his mother, a brother, and two aunts had all had pancreatic cancer. He feared it so much that he delayed being treated for a benign gastric ulcer.

Others have not had such a personal experience but have seen cancer statistics in the media and are extremely afraid of "learning the worst." They delay going to the doctor, even though most warning signs turn out not to be cancer. These feelings of fear, leading to the ostrich syndrome—wanting to put your head in the sand, thinking that the problem will just go away—can be both dangerous and foolhardy if the problem turns out to be cancer. As most people now know, a cancer diagnosed in the early stages is usually curable. So it is far better to overcome the fear or denial and see a doctor. The relief that follows finding out that it was nothing important allows life to get back to normal and the fears to be laid to rest. If the problem does turn out to be cancer, you will get a head start on the treatment and improve your chances of cure.

If you are putting off checking out a suspicious symptom because of anxiety, I strongly advise you to call your physician rather than letting your anxious feelings keep you from going through appropriate tests. Also, let your doctor know that you're having a lot of anxiety about what is happening and you may need help to control the fears, especially if difficult tests, like scans or sonograms, are ordered. If you have been troubled with anxiety in the past, or if you have feared cancer, it may be wise to ask your doctor for a referral to a mental health professional to help you get through the tests and procedures. The same advice holds for friends or loved ones who have these problems; you can play a pivotal role in ensuring they get help.

Before you go to the doctor, you may wish to make some notes to take with you so that you can give an accurate account of your symptom. You may also wish to have a family member or close friend accompany you, since it is sometimes hard to remember things when you feel nervous. Jack Price, a young man with melanoma, had thought about this issue when he told me this:

> *I think it's always helpful to have my wife in the room with the doctor for two reasons. One, because two people listen better than one. She picks up information I've completely overlooked. And two, I want her to be very much a part of the decision making.*

Once you have seen the doctor and had an examination, and the tests have been ordered—such as a biopsy, scans, or bone marrow aspiration—your thoughts may alternate between "It's probably nothing" and "I know it's the worst." Feelings of optimism and despair change from hour to hour. This is part of the response to the possibility of hearing bad news: anticipating what you may feel should it be cancer. Many people share with me that this is one of the most difficult times for them—waiting to hear the news.

Most tests today, including bone scans and sonograms, are generally performed on an outpatient basis rather than in the hospital, so it is good to take someone along to help you get home. You may not feel up to par if you're drowsy from medication that was given with the procedure. The diagnostic tests themselves may be difficult to tolerate if you have phobias—intense and overwhelming fears—of doctors, hospitals, needles, or seeing blood.

Judy was a young woman of thirty-five who had, since childhood, panicked when she had to go to the dentist or doctor. She was embarrassed that she often fainted at the sight of blood and when she had to have a blood test. Since she enjoyed good health, she was fortunate in having been able to avoid medical visits and hospitalizations so that her phobias rarely bothered her. When she found a lump in her breast, however, she had an anxiety attack, and when I saw her, all her old fears had returned "in spades." She couldn't sleep or eat during the week before her breast biopsy, which she managed to get through with the help of a prescription for the antianxiety drug clonazepam and much support from her boyfriend. The needle biopsy showed tumor cells. She was scheduled for a lumpectomy, and a small, 1.2-cm tumor was removed. Her anxiety diminished, and radiation therapy proved to be far less frightening, though she had some fears about the possible side effects. She described the brush with illness as a wake-up call to get a better handle on her problems, and she started psychotherapy to help her understand the origins of her fears.

If you have had fears of being confined in a small space (claustrophobia), you may find magnetic resonance imaging (MRI) to be frightening. This scan requires being placed in a small cylinder surrounded by a large, noisy machine. About 20 percent of people find it hard to tolerate, and about 5 percent are unable to go through with it. There are ways to make it easier today, such as listening to music or relaxation tapes or taking a medication to reduce your anxiety during the procedure. Tapes with instructions for relaxation, guided imagery, and meditation can be listened to ahead of time to help you become calmer (see Chapter 9). When you have an intense fear or phobia, it may seem so overwhelming that you cannot imagine overcoming it. But your doctor or a mental health professional can help you to relieve the fear to the point that you can get the medical tests you need.

The workup is important to determine the medical situation and to help you decide on a treatment course; therefore, any fears or phobias standing in the way must be looked into. Let your doctor know that you're frightened, that this fear has troubled you in the past; you can receive medication to be less anxious. Later, ask for a referral to a mental health professional to treat the phobia, so that you can get through future tests more easily.

THE DIAGNOSIS

> *The whole thing was like a bad dream, from the time the doctor gave me the diagnosis, till I started my treatment a few weeks later. I have no idea what I thought or felt or said or did. I was totally in a daze.*
>
> —Raymond, a retired businessman with lung cancer

Many people describe the period of waiting between hearing the diagnosis—the dreaded words "You have cancer"—and the start of their treatment as the worst time in their illness. The anxiety begins to peak when the bad news is given, but there isn't as yet any plan in place to move ahead and "fight it." It is difficult to tolerate the feeling that there are cancer cells in your body and nothing is being done to destroy them. The unspoken fear that "I might die" may seem more overwhelming when you are not yet receiving treatment.

This generalized anxiety can be compounded by worries about particular treatments. People worry about chemotherapy, for example, because they carry visions of chemotherapy as it was given twenty years ago, before drugs were available to control nausea and vomiting and other troublesome side effects.

Cornelius Ryan, famed reporter of the American forces' invasion of Europe in World War II, kept a diary of the time surrounding his diagnosis of prostate cancer in 1970. Ryan, who wrote the best-seller *The Longest Day,* dictated tapes that were his secret way of coping with the shock and the meaning of the diagnosis. He described in a masterly manner some of the emotions so many people feel.

> The diagnosis changes everything. . . . Now cancer will be my closest possession, going with me from office to house to conferences and dinner parties, as I go myself. I have got to get used to having it always here. I have got to think of what influence it may assume in time, not only over me, but on my family, friends and work. . . . What comes to mind immediately is how fast cancer alienates one from the usual routines and behavior. . . . It is odd that apart from a slight aching of the prostate . . . there is no pain, no dramatic change caused by this malignancy except in my mind. Does this cancer really exist? Did some harassed technician mix my slides with those of some other poor bastard's? . . . I am grasping at straws. I suspect it is not uncommon in the first few hours. There is simply no way to maintain a precise progression of thoughts and actions after such an emotional shock. My mind swings from disbelief to fatalism. I am vacillating between a surging belief that all will be well and a maudlin conviction that nothing will ever be right again. . . .
>
> Just now I thought of something that is probably the closest comparison to my present predicament I have ever experienced. During World War II, I found myself caught up in a patrol in a minefield. My reaction, and I remember it so well, had two distinct plateaus: how did I get myself into this situation? and, now, let's get out of it. Curiously, back then, I cannot remember experiencing fear. Neither do I recall any great surge of courage. I think my reaction was mechanical. There was no point in dwelling on the fact that we were in a minefield. The sole objective was to get through it safely—and somehow we did. . . . Now, as in those wartime days, I don't know what steps will bring me through this grave ordeal, but I can't stay rooted to one spot forever. . . . Without scientific knowledge to back me up, I would guess that the worst time emotionally is in the first few hours after you get the bad news.

Ryan says it all, in terms of those early responses to hearing the diagnosis. In other excerpts, he tells of his anger: "Why *my* body? Why *now* when I have so much to write?" Then he berates himself for his self-pity but retains his humor as a way of expressing the anger: "There's a mosquito in here buzzing around the desk. If it stings me, I hope the damn thing gets cancer."

Early in our work at Memorial Hospital, Dr. Mary Jane Massie and I tried to understand these first responses to a cancer diagnosis. People we talked with were responding in the same way that people do when faced with other kinds of catastrophic news—the death of someone close, a natural disaster such as an earthquake, or a personal catastrophe like the loss of a limb—that profoundly affect life and the future. We began to see a general pattern to hearing the bad news.

There is an initial response of *denial and disbelief.* "This can't be true! It's a mistake. I'm sure the slides sent to pathology were mixed up or the doctor confused my tests with somebody else's. It simply can't be happening to me." Ryan said it by suggesting that a harassed technician reversed the slides. Disbelief—"this couldn't be happening to me"—is probably the psyche's protective device to provide a little time and space to let the information "sink in," so that the person does not feel instantly overwhelmed.

We call the second stage the *turmoil phase.* The truth can't be denied; it *is* cancer. You begin to confront the reality more directly. This often creates a period of restlessness; fearfulness, which is hard to control; and preoccupation with the diagnosis and its implications. There is a sense of helplessness (What can I do?) and hopelessness (I can't find a way out), alternating with a sense of vague calm (Everything will be okay). Sleep may become erratic—eating may as well—and concentration on work and routine activities becomes impossible. You may repetitively go over all the fears that the word *cancer* conjures up: possible death with much pain, becoming disabled, perhaps needing surgery that will drastically change your body function or appearance, becoming dependent on others, losing the sense of acceptance from your family and friends, and then the terror of final abandonment. We know that these fears are exaggerated far beyond the actual likelihood of their happening. Still, they are powerful, as described so well by Ryan in his tapes. This stage often lasts a week or two, usually ending when you begin treatment and regain a sense of hope.

It is important to realize that this turmoil is a common, normal response to the threat to your life. You are not "going crazy." It is unfortunate that important decisions about treatment must be made during this time of high distress when thinking clearly is apt to be most difficult. Today, many people seek several opinions about what the best treatment might be, and the opinions are often different. Jack Price felt about his melanoma treatment that "surgeons are selling surgery; radiotherapists, radiation. . . . You know, it seems like the old saying that when you have a hammer in your hand, everything you see is a nail!"

Deciding whom to trust and with whom to cast your lot depends first on the treatment making sense to you, but also on finding a doctor you feel you can trust and who seems to have your best interests at heart. Your doctor should work in a hospital that has the necessary equipment and highly qualified staff to provide expert care for whatever complications may arise, as occasionally they do. It's good during this tough, stressful period to take one day at a time, make one decision at a time, and keep a clear head and calm mind. Because of the difficulty in processing information when highly stressed, you may wish to have a relative or close friend help you gather information, meet your doctor, and help you weigh your options.

This is a time when "browsing the Web" is tempting as a fast and easy way to get a lot of opinions. Chat rooms and websites have proliferated and have become a major source of uncensored information. Well-meaning friends often get into the act and offer options that raise anxieties but don't truly help in making decisions. Chapter 5 discusses working as a partner with your doctor and the role of the Internet. Facts from the Web should be seriously considered only after discussing the material with your physician.

A decision also has to be made quickly regarding whom you wish to tell your diagnosis, both in the family and outside. For some people, maintaining the aura of health is important for the financial or psychological well-being of others. They may find it difficult to make their illness public. Some of us recall the watershed events that led to drastic changes in social attitudes about cancer in the United States when Betty Ford, then the First Lady, made public her breast cancer and its treatment. Happy Rockefeller, Vice President Nelson Rockefeller's wife, did the same. It was suddenly okay to say you have cancer and to reveal the extent of it. They both announced that they would receive chemotherapy. A great deal of the stigma surrounding cancer, specifically breast cancer, was lifted. Today, an honest and open approach that reveals the diagnosis leads to the best opportunity for receiving the helpful support of others, although this attitude may be modified by personal style or circumstances.

Joanne, a fifty-year-old divorced economist, was diagnosed with lymphoma. She was the pillar of her family and her group at work as well. She found it difficult to tell anyone about her diagnosis and chose to go it in silence, cutting off the support from those she loved and who loved her the most. As she discussed her reasons, it became clear why she felt this way. She had experienced the death of her mother at a young age and immediately shouldered responsibility and tackled the adult issues of the household, including taking a job, delaying further schooling. In her family, you did not talk about problems, but simply accepted them silently and coped with them without complaining or bothering others. This pattern had served her well in her life in terms of coping, but it had a negative effect as she dealt with her diagnosis and her need to keep it a secret to protect others. She was the strong one in her family and could not relinquish the role. As we explored this lifelong pattern during some sessions of psychotherapy, she was encouraged to see that being strong in this situation required that she share the information with her daughter and son. They would be able to cope better with their concerns about her if they were "partners" and not left in the dark. Joanne also benefited from being open with her family, receiving their love and support as she underwent treatment.

The third stage of adjustment to the diagnosis usually comes when treatment begins, with the relief that comes from *doing* something about it. People usually feel reassured and become more optimistic as the treatment starts and they begin to work actively to combat the cancer and to return to their normal life. This is when we see the emergence of the many different ways people handle life's adversities. We enter into the realm of coping with disease and the broad range of coping styles developed by people on their own, honed by years of life experience.

As I discussed in my criticism of the current demands for "positive thinking," I have come to respect each individual's unique way of coping, and I try to help people find what works best for them in dealing with the crisis. Most studies, when you sum them up, suggest that what works best is dealing head-on with the issues of illness and treatment, seeing them as problems to be solved. This mind-set encompasses people who want to do extensive research to find the right doctor and treatment, as well as those who are content to move forward without getting more opinions, wishing to get on with the treatment as soon as possible. What we know doesn't work well, as mentioned earlier, is the ostrich syndrome: passively refusing to deal with the diagnosis realistically.

Jack Price was an A-plus active coper whom I came to know well, along with his wife and little girl. He was eager to tell doctors what it feels like to be ill, and both he and his wife spoke in seminars teaching our Fellows how to communicate better with patients. Jack had been cured of testicular cancer in his twenties and became a volunteer who talked with young people about cancer. He was unprepared as a thirty-four-year-old married man and the father of a two-year-old to find that he had malignant melanoma. As he said, "I had paid my dues already, how could this happen?" With an unusual form of melanoma for which no standard treatment existed, he described becoming "my own general contractor." He researched the Web ("working the catalogue," as he put it) and asked doctors to help him find centers around the country that were treating his condition. He tracked them down and made decisions with the help of a close doctor-friend. Difficult as it was, he coped best by taking an active approach after the diagnosis.

Jack Price, like Ryan, described how hard it was to believe he had a serious illness during those periods when he felt and looked healthy. He also was aware of how hard it was for others to believe that he had a serious illness, which, in turn, made it hard to talk about it. Jack had a wonderful description of how he felt, which I often use in helping other patients to understand the overwhelming and conflicting feelings they have as they sense their life is threatened:

> *Dr. Holland, I have these three gremlins in my head. One of them is on one side saying, "Jack, you're going to lick this—don't worry." Another gremlin is on the other side saying, "Jack, you dope, you know you aren't going to make it." And in the middle is this third little guy who has to make sense of both of them and help me to keep going on with my life day after day. Sometimes, they get so loud I can't think, but most of the time I keep them locked up, and when I'm busy they don't bother me.*

Surely, there are as many ways of coping as there are people, but the key is to be certain that the diagnosis doesn't paralyze you into inaction and the inability to seek treatment. Finding a doctor with whom you can talk comfortably and honestly and work as a partner is a key to success. When you connect with such a doctor, the two of you become a team; coping becomes easier because you have someone who will face the fears with you (see Chapter 5).

5

WORKING TOGETHER

If we want to avoid feeling tiny and powerless, we must take responsibility for our medical care where we can— with the medical professionals that we meet face-to-face.

—Carol Fernow, *Coach: How to Make the Human Connexion with Your Doctor*

Young physicians enter medical practice brimming with a mastery of medicine's vast technology, but sadly deficient in their ability to relate to the very people they have pledged to serve.

—C. Everett Koop, Chair, "Take Time to Talk," Advisory Council on Doctor-Patient Communication, 1998

For centuries, doctors had all the power in the patient-doctor relationship and patients had none. Beginning in the 1970s, patients gained the power and doctors had less and less. In the 1990s, both patients and doctors have lost their power. It has been taken over by third parties.

—Adapted from a lecture by Mark Siegler, M.D., physician and ethicist, University of Chicago

How did doctors become "providers," patients become "clients," and medical care, a "product"?

—Commonly heard from physicians

Doctors and patients alike are saddened and angered by the distance that increasingly interferes with their interaction. . . . As smaller and smaller players in ever growing

systems, both we who offer care and those who seek it too often keep a distance from one another. We doctors are told repeatedly how arrogant we appear, even as we ponder what is happening to the human side of medicine that attracted so many of us to medicine.

—Thomas Delbanco, *Annals of Internal Medicine,* 1992

And as I left his office, he said, "You know, you have a very bad disease, but we are going to take care of you." . . . I had full confidence in his expertise, his concern, and emotional support.

—A breast cancer survivor, quoted in the *Journal of Clinical Oncology,* 1999

*B*oth patients and doctors have expressed dismay at the way health care currently is delivered in this country, driven by market forces. The essence of health care has traditionally hinged on the personal relationship between a patient and a doctor, freely chosen by the patient to provide needed medical services. It's easy to sit and lament that the days of the home-visiting, hand-holding, kindly doctor carrying his black bag are gone. There was something comforting about seeing the physician arrive; he (it usually was a man) seemed like a living antidote against the fears of illness. Kindness, concern, and hand-holding were his most powerful tools. The black bag hardly carried any drugs that could cure an illness. Early in the twentieth century, Dr. Oliver Wendell Holmes is said to have remarked that "if the whole of the materia medica, as used now, could be sunk to the bottom of the seas, it would be the better for mankind—and all the worse for the fishes."

So be careful in wishing for the "good old days" of health care. The care might have been kinder and gentler, but the ability to diagnose and treat was primitive compared with today's remarkably sophisticated methods. The striking extension of the average length of life for both men and women is evidence of the success. Medicine has become increasingly "high-tech" in terms of tests to find out what is wrong. Hearing the patient's main complaint and the story of the illness and doing a physical examination form the cornerstone of making a diagnosis, but they are far from sufficient today. Blood tests, scans, and X rays all sharpen the accuracy of the diagnosis. But all these "smart tools" have had the effect of distancing the doctor from the patient and placing less importance on their interacting with each other. Increasing evidence suggests, surprisingly, that computers may be able to take diverse clinical information, process it, and come up with a more reliable diagnosis than the physician who is relying on clinical judgment alone.

In a medical equivalent of the Deep Blue versus Gary Kasparov chess contest, Lars Edenbrandt, an artificial intelligence expert at the University of Lund in Sweden, pitted a computer against a physician. Edenbrandt programmed the computer to "read" electrocardiograms (EKGs). He trained the computer by feeding it more than ten thousand EKGs, telling it which were from patients who had heart attacks. He then asked Dr. Hans Ohlen, an expert, to read several thousand EKGs and indicate which ones represented heart attacks. The computer rated the same EKGs—and won, with 20 percent greater accuracy.

What seems like a "bad news" story for the doctor-patient relationship may in fact have a silver lining. We can get greater accuracy and fewer errors in diagnosing diseases using technology, but there may be additional benefits. In a recent *New Yorker* article, describing this new computer capability with the potential to replace the fallible human being, Atul Gawande pointed out that in a new era "[physicians] will be freed to do what only *they* can do—talk to their patients. It's because medical care is about our life and death that we need doctors who can address our fears, hopes, and ignorance— doctors who can help give meaning to what we're going through."

It's not only high-tech diagnosis but also high-tech treatment that is changing medicine. Reflecting on my work with people with cancer, I have come to the view that the more high-tech the treatment a patient must go through, such as bone marrow transplantation or repeated cycles of high-dose chemotherapy, the greater the need for "high touch," since the emotional and human needs are greater. Fortunately, we have many ways to help you cope with your treatment today including many things that might be called high touch (described in Chapter 9).

In addition to the technological changes in medicine, health care in the United States has been turned on its ear in the past decade by managed care. The effect has been to batter the old-fashioned doctor-patient relationship. Health maintenance organizations (HMOs) and other managed-care plans reimburse physicians at such low rates per visit that doctors schedule shorter and shorter office visits in order to see more patients. Both patients and doctors decry the new order that speaks of vendors, customers, and products. Health care is something that was valued as somehow set apart from (and above) the world of business and the marketplace. Clearly, if patients and physicians banded together to protest, they could be more effective than either group could be alone. There is a need for new partnerships, between patients and physicians at a societal level.

These current problems point out even more emphatically how important the bond is between a doctor and a patient with cancer. My oncologist husband repeatedly mentions that "the mind is the only organ that is involved in every patient with cancer." He means the human dimension is the only aspect of cancer care that is involved in every encounter with every patient at every visit, no matter what the cancer diagnosis is or whether the treatment is surgery, radiation, or chemotherapy. You would think this fact would have gotten more attention in medical schools, especially regarding cancer, but it has been slow to be recognized. Medical schools are now beginning to provide doctors with training in how to give bad news. More effort is being made to teach the importance of communication and how to do it better. Patients and their families repeatedly stress the importance of the way the diagnosis is presented and how helpful it can be when it is told in a sensitive and kind manner.

Joan, a thirty-nine-year-old journalist, had her annual mammogram. The results were sent to her gynecologist, who called her and said, "I have the results of your mammogram, and I need to see you. We'll likely need to get a biopsy." Following the biopsy, she went back to her doctor, but this time Joan asked her husband to go with her because she had become increasingly anxious and worried, and she was not thinking as clearly as she usually did.

The doctor sitting with them said, "The biopsy confirms what I thought it might be. The spot on your mammogram (remember, you saw it, too?) is an early form of breast cancer. I know you must feel shaken, but we caught it early, and actually this type of cancer is highly curable. What we have to do is remove the lump first. Then we'll give some radiation to the breast, and after that, we may want to add chemotherapy."

Joan began to cry. "How can I deal with this now? I have my mother's illness and the children need me. Are you sure?" Her doctor told her he was certain of the diagnosis and that her distress was understandable. "Right now, the best thing for both of you is to go home," he suggested, "and take time to think this through. We can meet again in about a week and discuss a treatment plan." After a few days of worrying and sleeplessness, Joan called her doctor for an appointment to get more information and a clearer perspective: "How will you know if you've removed all the cancer? What will be the side effects of the radiation and chemotherapy?" Joan said her doctor answered her questions thoroughly, and she felt reassured enough to go ahead with her treatments.

A poignant story illustrates how important it is to give particularly bad news in the kindest way, told by a patient who experienced it both ways:

Warren, a thirty-eight-year-old lawyer, came to see me to ask advice about how to tell his family about his diagnosis of colon cancer. He had felt healthy and had no symptoms except for some rectal bleeding, which he initially had ignored after a physician erroneously told him that he had hemorrhoids without pursuing a proper diagnostic workup. Several months later, he found, to his astonishment, that he had colon cancer that had spread to his liver. He had small children, a young wife, an elderly father, and brothers. He had lost his mother to colon cancer several years earlier. After being stunned at the news that he had inoperable cancer, this young man asked the first doctor, who had made the diagnosis: "Tell me, man to man, how long do I have?" Without any discussion, the doctor replied coldly, "Three to six months," and walked out of the consultation room, leaving Warren alone to absorb the horror of what he had just heard. He told me that he felt like giving up there and then.

I suggested that he consult a liver surgeon, and he did. This doctor, a man in his sixties, talked with him and reviewed all the information. Afterward, this surgeon sat down, reached out to hold Warren's hand, and said, "Son, do you know how bad this is?" While the news was no better than it had been before, it was given in a compassionate and caring way, which he recalled with tears as he told me. The surgeon spoke with respect for his intelligence and feelings and made no guesses about time left, which are always unsure predictions. Warren continued to see the surgeon and decided to pursue aggressive treatment with chemotherapy and radiation, rather than just give up hope. He continued to feel well and was able to enjoy his time with his wife and children. He has survived for two years, already outliving the dire prediction given him so coldly.

You have a right as a patient to expect your doctor to be competent, to be assured that he or she is knowledgeable and technically skilled. However, you also have a right to expect caring and compassion from your doctor. Physicians who have these traits are able to think, "How would I want my doctor to treat me right now if I had received the same news?" Three C's form the cornerstone of good doctoring: competence, compassion, and caring.

A competent doctor without compassion or caring is daunting to the patient feeling uncertain and vulnerable. In diagnosing your cancer, your personal physician or general oncologist may say, in referring you to a specialist, "If I had this type of cancer, I would go with Dr. X." So you go to see Dr. X, reputed to be the expert or, if he or she is a surgeon, to have "good hands." And you may find that

Dr. X is very busy and keeps you waiting for quite some time, signs that this doctor is in great demand and, therefore, probably quite competent.

But when you finally get to see Dr. X, he or she is short with you, explaining matters in little detail and spending hardly any time with you. You may find yourself feeling "at sea," ill-informed, and ill at ease, at a time when you expect reassurance and hope to come away with confidence in the doctor. Clearly, you face a choice: You can say, "Competence comes first. I'll put up with the lack of emotional support." Or you can decide to seek another physician who is equally competent by reputation, but who puts caring into the paradigm by taking time to sensitively explain the treatment to your satisfaction.

Most young people go into medicine with a strong sense of humanity and humility, with the three C's strongly in place. But something happens to many in medical school as they cram in more and more facts: They become fatigued and think they lack time for considering the human side of illness. We speak of the first two years of medical school as "preclinical," when the basic sciences are studied, and the last two years as "clinical," when experiences with patients are the primary activity. Dr. Balfour Mount, physician and director of palliative care at McGill University, jokingly describes the two periods as the "precynical" and then the "cynical" years, reflecting this change in attitude. Fortunately, as clinical training advances, most doctors return to their humanism. Taking full responsibility for their patients leads them to a healthy recognition of how important compassion and caring are.

Lewis Thomas, physician–philosopher, suggested that every physician should have a serious bout of illness to see what it feels like to be placed in the care of strangers in a strange place, without your own clothes and belongings and with only a wristband to identify who you are. Most physicians who go through such an illness emerge with a new level of respect for their patients' point of view and for the importance of compassion and caring. Some medical schools have even had students become patients for a few days as part of their training, to allow them to get a feel of the vulnerability.

This concern for the human side of patient care is not new. In

November 1926, Dr. Francis W. Peabody, Professor of Medicine at Harvard and Director of the Thorndike Memorial Laboratory at the Boston City Hospital, gave a lecture entitled "The Care of the Patient," in which he described the philosophy of medicine he had pursued as a student, researcher, teacher, administrator, and physician. For him, the doctor-patient relationship could be successful only if the doctor was a *complete* physician, combining human qualities with scientific knowledge and approaching the patient as a total person who happened to be sick. Dr. Peabody told the following to students at the Harvard Medical School:

> *What is spoken of as a "clinical picture" is not just a photograph of a person sick in bed. It is an impressionistic painting of the patient surrounded by his home, his work, his relations, his friends, his joys, sorrows, hopes, and fears. . . . Thus the physician who attempts to take care of a patient while he neglects this [emotional] factor is as unscientific as the investigator who neglects to control all the conditions that may affect his experiment. . . . Treatment of disease immediately takes its proper place in the larger problem of the care of the patient. . . . The treatment of a disease may be entirely impersonal; the care of the patient must be completely personal. . . . One of the essential qualities of the clinician is interest in humanity,* for the secret of the care of the patient is in caring for the patient.

Less than a year following his lecture and its publication in the *Journal of the American Medical Association,* Dr. Peabody died at the age of forty-six. It became obvious that he had begun to lecture and write about the care of patients after he knew that he himself had cancer.

WHAT *YOU* CAN DO

So much for the doctor's perspective. What can *you* do to ensure that the human stage is set between you and the doctor so that you get the competent and compassionate care you want and deserve? Here are several points to keep in mind.

BEFORE THE VISIT: IDENTIFY THE MAIN PROBLEM

It is helpful to prepare for the visit by thinking through, or even writing down, what the main problem is that you have experienced. The doctor will call it your chief complaint (such as pain). Be ready to tell the first symptoms that occurred: "I was perfectly well until three weeks ago when I developed stomach pains. They have come and gone and I haven't been able to go to work." This tells the doctor rapidly how long you had the symptom, how severe it is, and that it is interfering with your activities.

KEEP A MEDICAL NOTEBOOK

It is important to have your information organized so that you can express it succinctly. I strongly suggest that you bring to all visits a small personal notebook in which you keep a record of prior doctors' visits, medicines you have taken, when X rays were taken, and test dates and results. Over the years, it is remarkable how hazy dates of tests and illnesses become. At Memorial Sloan-Kettering, patients are given a small notebook, called a Medical Passport. About the size of an official passport, it has a pocket inside for your health insurance cards, a list of your doctors' and pharmacy phone numbers, and any other information you need to keep readily available. Kept at home, this notebook helps you prepare for each visit to the doctor. For example, if you have been taking medicines prescribed by another doctor, you need to note the name and dose. Bring the bottle of pills along to the doctor's office to take the guesswork out of figuring out *exactly* what you have been taking; this eliminates the need to say, "You know, the little red pill," with all its potential for inaccuracy. Working together is the name of the game.

THE FIRST FIVE MINUTES

Your doctor may be absorbed in reading your file or may seem too hurried to respect the social amenities, so it may be helpful for you to set the stage, and greet the doctor, shake hands, and introduce yourself:

I'm Ms. _____, and I'm here to see you because of a
problem I've been having. It is a cough I've had for the past
three weeks, and I'm concerned about it.

Your preparation for the visit, as we have just discussed, will
make the first five minutes easier. Questions from the doctor will be
fewer when you have all the facts clear in your mind and can express
them succinctly. This short period often sets the stage for the quality of communication between you and your doctor. Mutual respect
is established, and you pave the way for confidence and trust in the
relationship.

DECIDE HOW MUCH INFORMATION YOU WANT

Because people have different personalities, they communicate
differently, and they need different amounts of information about
their illness. People who work in the communications field talk
about how individuals can be divided into "monitors" and
"blunters." The monitors are people who want all the facts and only
feel comfortable when they have them. This gives them a feeling of
being in control and lessens their anxiety. The blunters are people
who want to hear only what is necessary for them to know. Hearing
the facts that are not immediately relevant makes them more anxious
and contributes to a sense of being overwhelmed and out of control.
You may be like the monitors, who say up front, "I want to know
all the facts as they emerge. Don't keep anything from me." This
person may keep a chart of blood counts or a record of when a test
is due to remind the doctor in case he or she forgets. Some people I
have known recorded their test results on a chart so they could see,
for example, the course of changes in their PSA level (a marker for
prostate cancer). The doctor needs to recognize that you are one of
these people and should be willing to share the medical information,
almost like talking with a colleague. This partner dialogue is powerful and engenders respect and cooperation.

Jack Price, who was a quintessential monitor, said this:

Having confidence in the doctor is one thing, but having a good
working relationship is another. . . . It has to be a partnership.

Unfortunately, there's no consumers' guide to doctors. . . . I need to have information to make rational decisions. If you go to a financial planner, you aren't going to say, "Here's $100,000. Invest it for me," and then walk out of the room. You're going to sit down and say, "What are the options of places to put it? What kind of rate of return can I expect with each? What are the risks?" It's the same with patients—I want the same kind of thing—enough clinical information to make informed decisions about my treatment.

If you are a blunter, on the other hand, you may say, "I want to be part of this partnership, but I'm not the type who likes to follow my blood counts or PSA levels. I'll do better if you just tell me what I need to know. The overall picture is sufficient for me. The details upset me and make me worry a lot more." If you tell the doctor this, that you aren't a control freak who wants to know all, it will be easier for you and the doctor to communicate in the way you find best. Natalie Spingarn, a twenty-five-year survivor of metastatic breast cancer and author of the book *The New Cancer Survivors,* talks about "the right *not* to know." If you feel better dealing with the big picture and leaving the details to the doctor, that is as much your right as the right to full disclosure.

It is best simply to tell the physician up front which way you do best. The doctor will use this as a guide in talking with you.

CONSIDER HAVING SOMEONE THERE WITH YOU

Like some people, you may choose to be alone at doctors' visits so that whatever is said is kept confidential. Friends and family should respect this desire. Like others, however, you might find it helpful to have someone with whom you feel comfortable come along to the doctor's office or hospital to listen and discuss what went on. If you feel very ill, upset, or just plain shy, you may wish to have the friend or relative who accompanies you "advocate" for you with the doctor, to say for example, "My mother's very nervous about the surgery and hasn't been sleeping. Could you give her something to help her sleep?" There is no shame in asking someone to play this role, and it is quite common for a family member, such as a spouse, sibling, parent, child, or close friend to do so. It must, however, be your preference. Should the doctor suggest you speak privately, simply say, "I would like [my daughter] present. You can say anything you need to say in front of her."

EXPRESS YOUR CONCERNS

Your care has several different aspects: a rational, informational side; a technical side; and an emotional side. You must be able to express any of your concerns without feeling your doctor might regard them as inappropriate or foolish. You might hesitate to say, "I'm so nervous, I'm jumping out of my skin" or "I'm worried sick about what this diagnosis means for my children" because of the ethos that we must be strong. If sexual concerns are important to you, don't let embarrassment keep you from raising the topic. Keep in mind that sexual activity is normal and that doctors can discuss this without the social and personal overtones that keep you from talking about it with others. You must be assertive about bringing up any issues that are important to you without feeling inhibited. Asking for help or expressing your concerns and fears doesn't make you a "wimp" or emotionally weak, as discussed earlier.

Unfortunately, respect for this aspect of care still takes a backseat. Again, if you have to choose between a doctor who is competent and one who is caring, competence wins out for sure, and you look for your caring elsewhere. Marian, a sixty-year-old woman with cervical cancer told me this:

> I really can't stand my surgeon. He's rude and ill-mannered. He's not a warm person. But my doctor swears by him, and he seems to really know his stuff. So I figure, if this jerk keeps me alive, I'll get my emotional support from other people.

Nevertheless, you have a right to expect caring as well as expert care. Concern for the human side is not stated in the Patients' Bill of Rights, but it should be. (See the New York State Patients' Bill of Rights and statement of Patients' Responsibilities, given to patients at Memorial Sloan-Kettering Cancer Center and reprinted at the end of this chapter.)

If you feel that your doctor is ignoring your "human side," you may need to say so. Sometimes, the nurse picks up the slack and can give more time to listening and understanding problems. We count on the nurse, as part of the team, to pick up on problems that the physician may have missed. These experienced and highly trained nurses often make "telephone rounds" late in the day to check on patients. This proactive calling is reassuring to someone who is ill and lonely at home, especially if living alone.

WRITE DOWN YOUR QUESTIONS

Whether this is the initial visit with the doctor or a later visit, after you have had tests and are looking at treatment options, it is helpful to bring a list of questions that express your concerns. This again focuses the discussion on *your* concerns. The doctor may not raise these issues unless you do.

GET A SECOND OPINION

Many people are afraid of offending their doctor by saying that they want to seek a second opinion before they undertake a new treatment. This worry should not be a concern for you with a physician today. If your doctor is offended, that may tell you something that you need to know. Oncologists today encourage second opinions, and everyone gains confidence on hearing that a decision has been endorsed by another. Cancer is a disease for which the "first shot" is the most important, and you want to feel confident when you begin a treatment that it is, indeed, the one that offers the best outcome.

GET INFORMATION ON THE WEB

Doctors are getting accustomed to a new role as consultant to the patient who comes in armed with extensive information obtained "on the Web." Many reliable resources are available, like the websites of the National Cancer Institute and the American Cancer Society. You will find more information than you ever wanted when you start to search cyberspace to learn about your cancer and its possible treatments. The downside is that many of the sites are truly uncensored. You get information that's reliable sometimes and highly unreliable and erroneous at other times. The Internet is a remarkable resource, but what you learn should be carefully considered and discussed with your doctor, who can sort out the real from the unreal. I have seen people access information from the Internet about treatment protocols for a rare tumor that they would not have been able to obtain otherwise. But I have also seen patients devastated by reading dire statistics about a tumor, without the accompanying interpretation that would have been provided in a face-to-face discussion with a doctor. Use the Internet as a great source of information, but sift out the facts with a physician.

In summary, communication is a two-way process; you can control more of it than you think if you present your problems, thoughts, and wishes clearly, indicating whether you are someone who likes to have all the facts or just the facts needed to make decisions. Be organized and prepared to give the medical facts clearly, keep good records, ask all the questions you are concerned about, and make it clear that good communication, including attention to your emotional well-being, is essential to getting the care you want. Also make it clear that you will take responsibility to make that happen.

PATIENTS' RIGHTS AND RESPONSIBILITIES

Most states today have a Patients' Bill of Rights, which outlines what you can reasonably expect of the care in a hospital. For the state of New York, these rights are reproduced below. The Patients' Responsibilities, as presented at Memorial Sloan-Kettering Cancer Center, are also outlined following the Patients' Bill of Rights.

PATIENTS' BILL OF RIGHTS

As a patient in a hospital in New York State, you have the right, consistent with law, to:

1. Understand and use these rights. If for any reason you do not understand or you need help, the hospital must provide assistance, including an interpreter.

2. Receive treatment without discrimination as to race, color, religion, sex, national origin, disability, sexual orientation, or source of payment.

3. Receive considerate and respectful care in a clean and safe environment free of unnecessary restraints.

4. Receive emergency care if you need it.

5. Be informed of the name and position of the doctor who will be in charge of your care in the hospital.

6. Know the names, positions, and functions of any hospital staff involved in your care in the hospital and refuse their treatment, examination, or observation.

7. A no-smoking room.

8. Receive complete information about your diagnosis, treatment, and prognosis.

9. Receive all the information you need to give informed consent for any proposed procedure or treatment. This information shall include the possible risks and benefits of the procedure or treatment.

10. Receive all the information you need to give informed consent for an order not to resuscitate. You also have the right to designate an individual to give this consent for you if you are too ill to do so. If you would like additional information, please ask for a copy of the pamphlet "Do Not Resuscitate Orders—A Guide for Patients and Families."

11. Refuse treatment and be told what effect this may have on your health.

12. Refuse to take part in research. In deciding whether or not to participate, you have the right to a full explanation.

13. Privacy while in the hospital and confidentiality of all information and records regarding your care.

14. Participate in all decisions about your treatment and discharge from the hospital. The hospital must provide you with a written discharge plan and written description of how you can appeal your discharge.

15. Review your medical record without charge and obtain a copy of your medical record for which the hospital can charge a reasonable fee. You cannot be denied a copy solely because you cannot afford to pay.

16. Receive an itemized bill and explanation of all charges.

17. Complain without fear of reprisals about the care and services you are receiving and to have the hospital respond to you, and if you request it, a written response. If you are not satisfied with the hospital's response, you can complain to the New York State Health Department. The hospital must provide you with the Health Department telephone number.

18. Authorize those family members and other adults who will be given priority to visit consistent with your ability to receive visitors.

19. Make known your wishes in regard to anatomical gifts. You may document your wishes in your health care proxy or on a donor card, available from the hospital.

PATIENTS' RESPONSIBILITIES

This statement of Patients' Responsibilities was designed to demonstrate that we at Memorial Sloan-Kettering Cancer Center believe that mutual trust, respect, and cooperation are basic to the delivery of quality health care.

When you are a patient at Memorial Sloan-Kettering Cancer Center, it is your responsibility to:

1. Provide accurate and complete information about your past illnesses, hospitalizations, medications, and other matters related to your health.

2. Tell your physician or nurse if you do not understand your treatment.

3. Inform your physician or nurse if there is a change in your condition or if problems arise during your treatment.

4. Provide accurate information related to insurance or other sources of payment. Patients are responsible for assuring prompt payment of their bills. Tell us if you are having financial problems so that we may assist you in a timely manner.

5. Understand that it may become necessary to transfer you to another bed within the hospital.

6. Be courteous and considerate of other patients and of hospital staff. Patients are expected to assist

in maintaining a quiet environment and to be respectful of hospital property.

7. Honor our No Smoking policy.

8. Observe our visiting hours and inform your visitors of our policy.

9. Honor our check-out time on the day you are discharged.

COPING

I feel sometimes as if I'm caught in a gigantic bunch of moving gears. I panic for a minute . . . then take a deep breath and realize things aren't so bad. I'm actually coping well with a lot of stuff and the panicky feelings get back under control.

—Judy, a forty-year-old chef with leukemia,
reflecting on her early treatment

It is only in quite recent years that oncologists . . . have begun to confront squarely the emotional impact of [cancer and its treatment] and the fact that emotional states play a large role in the tolerability of treatment and, perhaps, in the outcome as well. . . . To many patients, stunned by the [cancer] diagnosis . . . it is like being trapped in the workings of a huge piece of complicated machinery.

—Lewis Thomas, M.D., physician-philosopher

For many people, a sense of relief accompanies starting treatment: "At last, I'm doing something to fight the cancer cells in my body." Your initial uncertainty and anticipation are over, and you have renewed hope and the feeling of getting back in control of your life.

Now begins the time of coping with the actual treatment. Waiting for your first treatment, you may feel a return of that fear of the unknown, which goes along with facing any new, unfamiliar, and potentially frightening experience. The "horror stories" we've all heard of how difficult cancer treatments were in earlier days can add to the fears. Surgery used to be more radical, meaning a bigger incision, more scarring, more pain, and a longer, more difficult recovery. Radiation doses were less controlled, causing more tissue damage, and chemotherapy was given without the medications that are used today to control the side effects of nausea and vomiting. One woman expressed it as, "Oh yes, I had the chemo-terror!" This fear of what's coming, which is often based on misinformation and misperceptions, can be greatly reduced by asking your doctor to walk you verbally through exactly what is going to happen, step by step, in advance, like a rehearsal for the main event. This exercise reduces stage fright, or "treatment fright." When you are well informed about what you will go through, you can mentally prepare yourself for each event, becoming less fearful and more self-confident about dealing with each.

WHAT MAKES COPING EASIER?

Several factors, we've found, tend to make coping with cancer and its treatment easier—or harder. Tables 1 and 2 outline the positives and negatives.

TABLE 1

FACTORS THAT CAN HELP YOU COPE

✓ Being a person who is . . .

Generally positive toward life

Able to take one day at a time

Optimistic and unlikely by nature to feel helpless during a crisis

Able to meet a challenge (like treatment) head-on

Not prone to become highly stressed in the face of challenges (treatment)

  Able to commit to a goal and "hang in" (fighting spirit)

  Able to see the humorous side of negative things ("black" humor)

✓ Having enough information about the treatment, its goals, and possible side effects

✓ Having a caring medical team that is supportive and reassuring

✓ Having a caring nurse who can interpret the doctor's communications

✓ Having support from others (family, friends)

✓ Having a belief system or philosophy of life that gives meaning to stressful situations

✓ Seeking counseling to change behaviors or ways of coping that are counterproductive

---

TABLE 2

FACTORS THAT CAN HINDER HOW YOU COPE

✓ Being a person who is . . .

  Generally negative toward life and its problems

  Unable to think one day at a time and worries about the future

  Pessimistic by nature and can easily feel helpless in the face of stress

  Apt to try to avoid a challenge when possible

  Prone to become nervous and distressed in the face of challenge

  Reluctant to persist in the face of stress and can easily become overwhelmed and feel hopeless

  Unable to see the funny side of a situation or to take oneself less seriously

✓ Feeling inadequately informed about the nature of the treatment: the need for it and its goals and side effects

✓ Having a medical team that communicates poorly and doesn't convey a sense of caring

✓ Feeling isolated, without a person with whom to share the stress

✓ Having no personal philosophy of life or belief system that gives you perspective on adverse events

PERSONALITY AND COPING

Personality is first and foremost. It is clear that certain personality and coping styles augur well for coping effectively with treatment. They are largely enduring qualities that one simply has or doesn't have. Each of us copes with crisis and adversity in a slightly different way, but if you tend to be optimistic in your outlook and to "see the glass as half-full" (or, even better, three-quarters full) rather than "half-empty," you're apt to be less distressed and less likely to anticipate the worst. People cope better when they face a problem or crisis head-on, rather than try to avoid the inevitable or count on its going away (the old ostrich syndrome again). Successful copers tend to feel challenged rather than thrown or defeated by a problem, and they believe they can master it. They also demonstrate a "fighting spirit," committing themselves to a goal, hanging in, and following through.

Don't despair if you weren't born with these traits. Your cancer doesn't know it. Your personality traits affect how you behave, not how the cancer behaves. Some people seem to be born pessimistic, just as others seem like born alarmists or complainers; that's how they see the world and it's how they let off steam. People with these so-called negative characteristics can also get through cancer and survive it well. If you fall into this category or find it hard to hang in through tough times, you need to compensate by getting extra support from friends, family, your oncology team, or a counselor. Talking with a cancer survivor who has gone through the same treatment can be helpful; someone who is living proof that you can make it becomes a beacon of hope. Practical advice from survivors has a credibility that other people's advice lacks, because you know they have been there. Many hospitals and cancer centers have peer counseling programs, in which survivors of the same cancer you have are available to talk with you about what to expect as you go through treatment. If no such program is available, ask if you can talk with someone who has had the same cancer you have.

If you have traits that might lead to poor coping, it is important to be alert early in your treatment to how you are doing. Ask for help, since some of these negative coping styles can be turned around, making it easier for you to go through your treatment. Psychological help is available through individual sessions or in groups with other cancer patients (see Chapter 9). Both are aimed at reducing distress, which is often relieved just by sharing your feelings about your illness and treatment with someone who listens and understands.

YOUR BELIEFS

Having or developing a philosophy of life or a belief system can give you a perspective for going through treatment in a way that makes it easier for you to tolerate the rough spots. Barbara White Fishman, artist and philanthropist, put it this way:

> For me, knowing that I was seriously ill opened doors and opportunities that have truly enriched my life. It is through cancer that I have rediscovered my love of painting and refocused my energies to help others. Both have given me tremendous strength and satisfaction. There is a positive side in that cancer often serves as a wake-up call that life is precious and each moment should be appreciated.

Another person told me:

> *I would not have taken time to discover who I am and what*
> *life is about if I hadn't developed cancer. It sounds strange but I*
> *consider it a gift from God.*

Some other factors are harder to control, since they're not personal factors, but they count strongly in making coping with treatment easier. Feeling you understand the reason for the treatment, its goals and side effects and the other options available to you, makes it easier to stay the course and keep a rational approach, especially when it gets rough. For example, you might feel like throwing in the towel if your first chemo treatment leaves you feeling wiped out. But if the doctor explains that only a complete cycle of chemo treatments can give you the best chance of getting rid of your cancer, you will probably find the resolve to do whatever is needed to try to "beat it."

Troubling side effects such as hair loss from chemotherapy become easier or at least possible to bear if you can "keep your eye on the ball" in terms of the trade-off between short-term side effects and the possibility of long-term benefit and survival. As long-time lung cancer survivor and writer Alice Trillin put it, "I told the doctors, I don't care about my hair. I want to be a grandmother."

Of course, understanding and being committed to the treatment are inseparable from finding a caring doctor and health care team with whom you feel confident and who are "there for you." Having a close friend or loved one who shares the burden of treatment is another positive. Many people must manage alone, because they lack a close family member or friend, and they *do* manage, but it may be harder. These individuals may find a support group particularly helpful, since the bonds that form among group members often become a substitute for absent significant others or family. Some people want to shield those close to them. For them, the groups become a safe place to talk. (Chapter 9 provides more information about groups.)

SENSE OF HUMOR

One helpful trait is the ability to "lighten things up" by putting difficult situations in a humorous perspective. It isn't easy to laugh when you don't feel good, but lots of evidence shows that being able to laugh at yourself and the situation is helpful and good for you. Norman Cousins popularized the idea, by claiming that watching funny movies (he watched Marx Brothers movies) helped him sleep pain-free, despite a painful, degenerative arthritis-like condition. Mind-body, or psychoneuroimmunology, research backs up his claim. At the Loma Linda University Medical Center in California, Dr. Lee S. Berk and his colleagues found that laughter lowers the level of stress hormones (natural substances in our bodies that we release when we are stressed). I see humor being used over and over again as a way to take the sting out of a thoughtless comment, to laugh at one's own reaction, or to tolerate a particularly difficult time.

We often refer to this kind of joking as "black humor" or "gallows humor": putting a funny spin on a painful, serious situation. It is used by medical teams and is regarded as a critical balancing tactic for interns and house staff who are stressed, fatigued, and pushed to the max. I often call this the "MASH mentality," reminiscent of the MASH frontline hospital unit portrayed in the long-running TV show. People slog through extreme circumstances by joking, making the best of what can't be changed, and finding an unusual closeness to others going through the same experience.

We also see this phenomenon among patients. Humor in the face of adversity seems to inspire an esprit de corps that contributes to greater coping and closeness.

New York Times columnist Robert Lipsyte, a testicular cancer survivor, calls this "tumor humor," a form of joking that I hear repeatedly. Here are some samples of tumor humor:

William Matthews in a poem in the *Atlantic Monthly* noted:

> *Once you've had cancer, you don't get headaches anymore,*
> *you get brain tumors, at least until the aspirin kicks in.*

Betsy, a woman of fifty-four, had just completed chemotherapy for breast cancer. She was returning to her normal life when a mammogram revealed something in her treated breast. She described her reaction with a smile that expressed the irony and the pain:

> When my doctor said, "We have to start treatment for a second tumor in your breast," I said, "That's impossible, I already gave at the office."

A man with lung cancer chose humor as a way of dealing with his children, who were devastated by his having chemotherapy and losing his hair. He teased them by saying:

> But don't you see? Everybody worries about getting cancer. I don't have that worry anymore—I've got it!

Humor can be a great way of dealing with the "dumb" comments from others when you are going through treatment for cancer. Several people have expressed with good humor their reaction to friends' comments on how "well you look," which makes them worried that either the friend is lying or they really look awful or they must have looked horrible the last time their friend saw them. One person quipped:

> The best thing about cancer is that people keep telling you how good you look, but that's when I really start to worry.

Another woman with lung cancer described to others in a lung cancer support group how a good friend had treated her, seemingly unaware of the contrasting situations. While not an example of the use of humor, her reaction demonstrates a good-natured recognition of an ironic situation:

> My friend had to have a breast biopsy. She was scared to death and needed a lot of support and asked me to go with her. When the procedure was over and the biopsy was negative and she

*was fine, she started to lecture me on how I have to be strong to
cope with my lung cancer treatment. I wanted to hit her.*

ONE DAY AT A TIME

One way we differ, which affects coping, is how we view time and
the future. The diagnosis of cancer creates a sense of urgency about
time that goes along with the uncertainty it causes. However, the person who can say "I'm just going to take one day at a time" is able to
stay focused on the tasks of that day. The person who hardly enjoys
today because of concerns and worries about tomorrow has a much
harder time dealing with illness. I often remind people that you can't
live yesterday or tomorrow, only today. William Osler called it "living
your life in day tight compartments." Any big task seems overwhelming until you break it down into manageable parts. The Chinese say,
"You move a mountain by moving one stone at a time." Hard as it is
to keep thinking that way, coping with cancer is easier if you try not
to focus on all the challenges that may lie ahead, but rather, stay
focused on today, during which you can accomplish something
despite the problems caused by the treatment.

DO'S AND DON'T'S FOR COPING WITH CANCER

The following do's and don't's are intended to be commonsense
guidelines to help you avoid feeling "trapped in the workings of a
huge piece of complicated machinery." I developed these "Holland's
homilies," as my staff calls them, from working with people with
cancer. They incorporate my ideas about the tyranny of positive
thinking and how to deal with some of the attitudes that are out
there about coping with cancer, some of which, as we described in
Chapter 2, create more problems to deal with.

1. DON'T believe the old adage that "cancer equals death." There are eight million survivors of cancer in the United States today.

2. DON'T blame yourself for causing your cancer. There is no scientific proof linking specific personalities, emotional states, or painful life events to the development of cancer. Even if you may have raised your cancer risk through smoking or some other habit, there is no benefit to blaming yourself or beating yourself up.

3. DO rely on ways of coping that helped you solve problems and handle crises in the past. If you've been a talker, find someone with whom you feel comfortable talking about your illness. If you're an inveterate nontalker, you may find relaxation, meditation, or similar approaches helpful. The secret, however, is this: Use whatever has worked for you before, but if what you're doing isn't working, seek help to find other ways to cope.

4. DO cope with cancer "one day at a time." The task of dealing with cancer seems less overwhelming when you break it up this way, and it also allows you to focus better on getting the most out of each day, despite illness.

5. DON'T feel guilty if you cannot keep a positive attitude all the time, especially when you don't feel good. Low periods will occur, no matter how good you are at coping. There is no evidence that those periods have a negative effect on your health or tumor growth. If they become frequent or severe, though, seek help.

6. DON'T suffer in silence. Do use support and self-help groups if they make you feel better. Leave a group that makes you feel worse, but don't try to go it all alone. Get support from your best resources: your family, friends, doctor, clergy, or those you meet in support groups who understand what you are going through.

7. DON'T be embarrassed to seek counseling with a mental health professional for anxiety or depression that interferes with your sleep, eating, ability to concentrate, or ability to function normally if you feel your distress is getting out of hand.

8. DO use any methods that aid you in getting control over your fears or upset feelings, such as relaxation, meditation, and spiritual approaches.

9. DO find a doctor who lets you ask all your questions and for whom you feel mutual respect and trust. Insist on being a partner with him or her in your treatment. Ask what side effects you may expect and be prepared for them. Anticipating problems often makes it easier to handle them if they occur.

10. DON'T keep your worries or symptoms (physical or psychological) secret from the person closest to you. Ask this person to accompany you to visits to the doctor when treatments are to be discussed. Research shows that people often don't hear or absorb information when anxious. A second person will help you interpret what was said.

11. DO reexplore spiritual and religious beliefs and practices such as prayer that may have helped you in the past. (If you don't consider yourself a religious or spiritual person, garner support from any

belief system or philosophy that you value, such as humanism.) These beliefs may comfort you and may even help you find meaning in the experience of your illness.

12. DON'T abandon your regular treatment in favor of an alternative or complementary treatment (see Chapter 10). Use alternative treatments that do no harm and that can safely be used along with your regular treatment. Be sure to tell your doctor which complementary therapies you are using or want to use, since some should not be used during chemotherapy or radiation treatments. Discuss the benefits and risks of any alternative or complementary treatments with someone you trust who can assess them more objectively than you when you are under stress. Psychological, social, and spiritual approaches are helpful and safe, and doctors encourage their use today.

13. DO keep a personal notebook with all your dates for treatments, laboratory values, X-ray reports, symptoms, and general status. Information is critical in cancer treatment, and no one can keep it better than you (see Chapter 5).

THE CONTINUUM OF DISTRESS: WHEN TO REACH OUT FOR HELP

How well or how poorly you are coping at a particular time contributes to your level of emotional distress. Distress is a broad term that describes the unpleasant emotions that occur normally with cancer. Virtually every person confronted with the diagnosis and treatment feels vulnerable and sad about the loss of health and the sense of well-being. It is normal to feel uncertain and worried about the future. But an important question that arises is this: When does the distress become so great that it falls beyond the acceptable range so that you need professional help?

Sadness is the "normal" end of one continuum that goes all the way to serious depression, which can become so severe that you find it impossible to enjoy the things that you ordinarily enjoy. If you are depressed, you may feel helpless and hopeless, overwhelmed, and unable to eat, sleep, or concentrate. At its worst, you can't get out of bed, carry on work or daily activities, or get yourself to the next treatment. The depression, then, is having an effect on your ability to continue your cancer treatment.

Anya, who had had several depressions before developing ovarian cancer, told me, "Cancer is not nearly as painful and hard to deal with as the depressions I've had in the past. I'm afraid, if my depression comes back now, I really won't be able to cope." We worked on preventing Anya's depression from coming back, recognizing that she was particularly vulnerable to it during illness. The "double whammy" would be too much for her to bear.

Your normal fears and worries, too, can spiral into a severe anxiety reaction, with panic attacks, phobias, tension, and distress. The distress may be barely tolerable, keeping you awake at night, robbing you of your appetite, and making you feel restless, frightened, and irritable. If you were a nervous person before, or had phobias, you are more likely to develop severe anxiety symptoms during illness. In cancer, these two emotions, worry and sadness, occur together, constituting most of the emotionally distressing side of cancer. Both can become more severe, but they are not a sign of mental illness or personal weakness. In a study done in 1984 in three cancer centers, just over half of the patients interviewed had distress that was severe enough to warrant further evaluation and treatment. The distress experienced by most of these individuals (about two-thirds) was caused by dealing with cancer, but the remaining third had some prior psychological problem, such as a phobia, that made it harder for them to deal with their illness.

A simple test is to rate how distressed you are on a scale of 1 to 10 (1 being no distress at all, and 10, severe distress). If you rank your distress from 1 to 4, you are probably doing just fine. If it is 5 or higher, you could benefit from extra support. However, if you rate your distress as 8, 9, or 10, and particularly if you have been feeling low, highly nervous, or scared over several days, call your doctor right away for a referral to a counselor or therapist who has experience working with people who have cancer.

A common problem for cancer patients with intense anxiety or depression is that their oncologist often doesn't recognize it, so that they don't get the counseling they need. About one out of every three people treated in oncology clinics is highly distressed, but surprisingly, less than one out of ten gets referred for help. One has to ask why? It is disappointing that while the stigma of cancer is diminishing, the stigma surrounding psychological and psychiatric problems is still widespread. People often suffer in silence rather than tell their doctor that they are having a hard time coping. Some attitudes that keep patients from speaking up are embodied in comments I've heard such as these:

- *I'm too embarrassed to tell my doctor about my problem. (This is especially true if it's a sexual problem.)*

- *He'll think I'm a wimp and maybe won't take care of me.*

- *They'll think I'm crazy.*

- *My cancer problem is real—what could psychological help do for me?*

- *She'll think I complain too much.*

- *He'll tell me that the most important thing is to get the cancer to shrink, not to get sidetracked.*

- *My family relies on me to be strong. If they think I'm having a hard time, they'll all fall apart.*

These attitudes, sadly, often prevent people from getting the help they need.

I've also heard doctors admit that they are reluctant to ask about psychological problems because "I'm not trained to handle them, and if I ask, it'll take all day. I'll be opening Pandora's box." Some doctors even believe the patient will be angry if asked about emotional problems. The net result is a "don't ask, don't tell" policy, like the one President Clinton chose to use in handling gays in the military. This approach has not worked well in the military, and it doesn't help in patient care either. In addition, shorter visits (increasingly mandated by the unfortunate realities of managed care) don't lend themselves to exploring the human side of care.

These barriers are best overcome by your pointing out that your cancer care must include concern for you as a person, not just treatment of your tumor. Because most causes of distress relate to illness, such as a need to understand better your medical condition, the treatments available, and "what to expect" in general, your doctor is the best person to deal with these concerns. The oncology nurse or social worker often can provide additional information. Many people welcome this "two-tier approach" because the nurses and social workers on the oncology team with the physician are good, interested listeners who don't convey the sense of being rushed.

Steve and Louise, a couple in their forties, were highly terrified that the cancer had returned a year after Steve was treated for prostate cancer. Both his father and grandfather had died of the same cancer. Steve became extremely nervous when his family doctor noticed a "shadow" on his hipbone X ray. He returned to his oncologist for a consultation on the matter. The oncologist gave them a clear explanation of the biology of prostate cancer, drawing diagrams to illustrate that the shadow was an old scar from an old break. It was *not* related to the prostate cancer, which had not returned. They were reassured and their anxiety level dropped with a sigh of relief. The explanation of the medical facts was sufficient.

If the problems or worries related to your illness, or even other worries, are occupying your mind a lot of the time or feel too intense for you to manage on your own, then it is important that you get the name of a mental health counselor with experience in cancer from your oncology team.

WHAT PROBLEMS REQUIRE PROFESSIONAL HELP?

FEELING OVERWHELMED BY FEAR AND DISTRESS

Intense worry about what cancer will do to you and its threat to your future and that of your family can shake the heartiest among us. In this situation, you feel a mix of anxious and depressed feelings that get in your way to the extent that you are barely able to carry on your work, take care of yourself and your family, and take care of your home—in short, to engage in your basic daily activities.

In today's fast-paced and highly stressed world, many people feel that they are barely able to keep their heads above water, juggling the normal concerns of work, family and other relationships, household, and finances. Suddenly, along comes cancer, which throws a wrench into the works. You may want to say "Stop the world, I want to get off," to borrow the title of the Broadway musical, but life doesn't work that way. So while you schedule your chemo or radiation sessions or need time to recover from surgery, the kids still need to be fed, picked up at school, and dropped at the baby-sitter; the dog has to be walked; the bills still have to be paid (and now there are medical bills on top of the usual ones); and on and on. And you might feel lousy or exhausted to boot. The straw that breaks the camel's back may be enough to send a champion coper into a tailspin, feeling you just can't cope with anything else.

It is important to recognize that this, too, shall pass. But it is also essential to get the help you need. I am always moved by the stories of friends, relatives, and neighbors who carpooled the kids to school, cooked food for the family, and came to the hospital. "I never could have made it without my friends," said Vicki, a forty-five-year-old single mother with breast cancer. "When I finished my chemo, I threw them all a big party."

In addition to helping you put your fears and sadness in perspective, counseling can help you manage these crises and solve the domino effect that cancer may trigger.

A PREVIOUS HISTORY OF EMOTIONAL PROBLEMS

If you have previously had to deal with anxiety, such as a phobia of needles, hospitals, or seeing blood, or if you have had agoraphobia—a fear of leaving home—you may be more troubled and emotionally upset by thoughts of going through treatment for cancer. Even the tests to diagnose cancer, such as CT scans, MRIs, and sonograms, are frightening to some people. The hospital visits and all the travails that the treatments entail are frightening in themselves and add to the ordinary burden imposed by this serious illness. If you have had panic attacks under stress in the past, or if you are a generally nervous, anxious, and fearful person, you may need help.

If this is your pattern, it is best to preempt the problem and seek help before it arises so that it doesn't interfere with your cancer treatment later. Discuss this concern with both your oncologist and your psychiatrist. Both physicians should be aware of all the medications you are taking (including any alternative or complementary treatments) so that drug interactions can be avoided. Together, you and your doctors can develop a treatment plan.

WHEN TREATMENT SITUATIONS PROVOKE ANXIETY

John, a sixty-year-old taxi driver, became nervous anytime he felt something was wrong with his body. He had always feared cancer, and he often went to the doctor with symptoms that were not serious. His wife teased him by calling him a hypochondriac. At an annual checkup, he was found to have an elevated level of prostate-specific antigen (PSA), which is a blood test that is used to screen for prostate cancer. Although his PSA level was elevated, he had no signs of cancer, so his doctor recommended "watchful waiting," with repeat PSA tests every three months to see if the level would rise. This approach provoked high anxiety, particularly just before each test. This "PSA anxiety" is common, but it is greater in those with a preexisting tendency toward anxiety (or, at its extreme, panic). John's doctor referred him

to my office for a consultation. We discussed his long-standing problems with anxiety, which had largely been tolerable;
but now the week before each PSA test was hellish for him.
He would be awake all night, unable to sleep, and would
constantly be so distracted by worries throughout the day
that he couldn't even go to work. Driving in traffic was
impossible for him.

We agreed that the week before the test he needed to
take medication at bedtime to ensure his rest and that a low
dose of an antianxiety drug during the day would reduce his
constant worrying. On this regimen, he managed to work
during the week before his doctor's visit. After the test was
over and the nurse called to give him the reassuring results of
the test, he would stop the medication for two months until
the week before the next PSA test, when he would start taking his medication again. In between these periods, we met
regularly to help him understand his longer-term problems
with anxiety and the nature of his fears of illness.

Some people have been vulnerable to episodes of depression all
their life. Developing a serious medical condition can bring depression back. We've said that it's normal to be sad when you're sick, but
clinical depression is an illness of its own, and it can be fatal, through
its risk of suicide. Professor Lewis Wolpert, in his book *Malignant
Sadness*, wrote:

> *Depression is sadness that has become pathological. Just as can-
> cer is a normal growth process that has gone out of control, so depres-
> sion is a normal emotion that has become viciously disordered.*

I saw a man of forty-five, Victor, who had finished treatment for lymphoma and was considered medically well and
likely cured. He had had a bout of depression in his thirties
following a divorce but had managed for years to be free of
its grip. Now, however, despite the good news, he found
himself choosing to spend his nights alone. He was an avid
reader and loved classical music, but he couldn't pay atten-

tion to what he was reading and he couldn't listen to music; not only did he not enjoy it, but it upset him more. At the office, he couldn't stay focused on his work. Sleep was fitful, and he had no desire for food. Victor's friends noticed that he wasn't himself.

Luckily, Victor was referred by his hematologist for evaluation of his depression. Victor told me his symptoms in a listless, dejected way, recalling his prior depression, which had been successfully treated with medication and psychotherapy. He told me that his brother had had severe depression and committed suicide. Also, his father had been depressed in his later years. Victor recognized his own vulnerability related to this family history. We started the antidepressant sertraline (Zoloft), to which he responded well in a couple of weeks, but we continued to meet over the following months to be sure that his early improvement continued.

A RECENT PERSONAL LOSS

Dealing with cancer is hard enough when other things are all right, but it becomes much more difficult to bear if you are grieving from the death of someone very close to you. (Chapter 16 deals with grief in more detail and what can be done for it.) It can be crucial to get help to deal with this "double whammy" to prevent serious depression and to keep you from giving up and not pursuing your recommended course of treatment. Grieving for a loved one while you're dealing with your own illness may lead to more thoughts about death. Under these circumstances, suicidal thoughts are more common and suicide is a higher risk. It is a good idea to seek a consultation with a mental health professional and share these thoughts. It is possible that grief counseling may be sufficient, but psychotherapy and a medication may be required to address the problem. In any case, persistent suicidal thoughts are not normal, and they should be a wake-up call to consult with someone. They are of serious concern and should be explored with a professional right away.

WHEN PARENTS OR OTHER FAMILY MEMBERS HAVE DIED FROM CANCER

The diagnosis of cancer can bring back memories of living through the illness and death of a loved one, and it may evoke the fear that you will suffer the same fate.

Sharon was a youngster of eleven when her father was diagnosed with bladder cancer. Her dad was an invalid at home for five years and died when Sharon was sixteen. Her childhood was colored by her father's illness and death. Her own diagnosis of ovarian cancer occurred at age thirty-six, when her children were ten and eight. She sought help to deal with her fearfulness, sadness, and recurring nightmares, which were about caring for her father. She recalled this childhood experience vividly and told me in detail about how difficult it had been for her as the oldest child. She related these memories to her own illness and realized how much she feared the same loss could happen to her children, whom she desperately wanted to protect.

Sharon came to see me once a week for six weeks, during which time she recounted these early experiences and how they had come to haunt her since her cancer was diagnosed. She rationally recognized that the doctor had assured her that her cancer was caught early and that she should be fine. She began to practice meditation daily for twenty minutes, which further added to her sense of control. We were able to see that her real concern was her identification with her two children and her anguish, as she imagined they might have to go through the same experiences as she did in childhood. Her anxiety went down to tolerable levels, and she phones occasionally to report that she is coping well.

MEMORIES OF A MAJOR TRAUMA EARLIER IN LIFE

A cancer diagnosis often ignites memories of traumatic events from the past that have been kept out of consciousness successfully for years. Suddenly, flashbacks and profoundly disturbing memories are rekindled: of combat experiences with their sense of vulnerability, fear, and death; of repressed experiences of childhood abuse; of World War II experiences in concentration camps, where the sense of helplessness, panic, despair, and death prevailed; of being trapped in a natural disaster, such as an earthquake, hurricane, or flood. Memories are frequently revived under the stress of dealing with cancer. These symptoms represent posttraumatic stress disorder (PTSD), in which the current trauma triggers memories of an earlier trauma, with renewed anxiety, depression, flashbacks, and overall distress (Chapter 11 covers PTSD in more detail).

It's quite common, also, for news events of a sad or tragic nature to transiently increase fears, distress, and sadness. When Jackie Onassis died of lymphoma, there was a torrent of emotion from patients who were struggling with their own cancer illness. Some followed the story in newspapers or magazines and on TV, and they cried for her and for themselves. Others couldn't read or watch what was happening; they felt too sad.

The death of Princess Diana in August 1997 held many around the world dazed and bound to the images that came through the news. Hundreds of millions of people followed her funeral on TV. Universally, people felt empathy, sadness, and a sense that the days around her death and funeral were like a personal tragedy. Even more recently, the untimely deaths of John F. Kennedy Jr., his wife, and his sister-in-law led to a similar outpouring of emotions. People who were grieving or who themselves were ill said to me, "I just had to turn off the TV; I couldn't watch it. It's just too sad and depressing for me to see that happening right now."

For people with cancer, the identification with a celebrity or a public figure who is ill or has died may carry an added meaning. It leads to the thought "if Jackie Onassis's illness could take a sudden turn for the worse, so could mine." The empathy for, or identification with, another can ignite fresh concern and preoccupation with illness and death. For most people, the uncertainty surrounding cancer never fully goes away, and these flashpoints simply bring it to center stage. Given a little time, distress related to the sad events in the news will recede into the background, and life and illness will feel manageable once more.

SUDDEN CHANGE IN MOOD OR MENTAL FUNCTION DURING CANCER TREATMENT

Some anticancer medications, particularly corticosteroids (also called steroids), interferon, pain medicines, and others, can cause a sudden, radical change in mood, mental function, and behavior. Families often react, saying, "Oh, his cancer is getting him down, he's so depressed." But when you look a bit more closely, it is clear that the change is due to a side effect of a medication (see Chapter 7). Indeed, a patient with cancer may become confused and unable to think clearly, entering a state of delirium, in which the brain is taking a hit from some toxic factor or event. The person may become confused about where he or she is and develop hallucinations, delusions, and fears of being harmed by someone.

Fran, a well-adjusted woman of sixty-five, came to the hospital for treatment of a painful spinal cord tumor. She was given steroids to reduce the pressure in her spine. On the third day, her family members were astounded when they came to visit her. She was terrified and told them, "There are people outside selling drugs, and the police are coming to bust me—save me!" Her adult children reported her reaction to her doctor, who explained that it was due to the high dose of steroids she was given. Her steroid dose was lowered and she was given olanzapine (Zyprexa) to reduce her frightening ideas. She soon became herself again, but she vividly remembered the strange feelings that were so alien to her. She commented, "I'm so glad to learn it was a drug that made my brain play tricks on me, and I'm not going crazy."

PHYSICAL SYMPTOMS CAUSING DISTRESS

Almost any pain in the body is made worse when we are anxious, and this is especially true for people with cancer, whose first fear on feeling a pain is that their cancer has spread. Patients who have pain will likely require medicines to control it, but psychological support, behavioral techniques (such as relaxation), and spiritual practices (such as meditation) can help a lot (see Chapter 9).

Nausea and vomiting from chemotherapy are remarkably better controlled today by antinausea drugs, which make it far easier to go through chemotherapy. However, anxiety about chemotherapy can increase the nausea and distress. People can even develop nausea just by thinking about the next treatment. This form of anxiety, an anticipatory symptom, is a kind of self-fulfilling prophecy. Scientifically, we understand it as a learned or conditioned response, like that of Pavlov's dogs, who reflexively salivated at the sound of a bell. Repeated chemotherapy treatments can trigger anticipatory nausea based on previous experience; the person expects it to happen so strongly that it does, in fact, occur before the stimulus is given. Reducing anxiety through a relaxation exercise, meditation, or an antianxiety medicine can eliminate this psychological side effect (see Chapter 9).

Fatigue and its causes are far better understood these days, and far more is being done about the problem. It is a cardinal symptom of which many patients complain. Fatigue affects three-quarters of patients with cancer at some time. It can range from having less energy than usual to finding yourself too exhausted to get out of bed or carry out the ordinary tasks you are used to doing every day. Some people say, "Just lifting my finger is an effort." And it can last from a few days to months. Fatigue can be caused by the cancer itself, by anemia, by treatments (particularly radiation and chemotherapy), by pain medications, or by depression. Tell your doctor about your fatigue so that its severity can be evaluated and its cause determined. Anemia can be treated and depression can be alleviated. Drugs called psychostimulants counter fatigue and improve energy levels. (see Chapter 9).

Insomnia, which can involve trouble going to sleep, awakening during the night, or awakening too early in the morning, is a common complaint that makes it harder to cope with the daytime stresses of cancer. Surely, nighttime is when "demons" and fears are apt to be on the loose, keeping you awake and allowing frightening thoughts to take over. Patients who aren't sleeping become more fatigued and overwhelmed, so that coping becomes more difficult. Reading, meditation, or listening to relaxation tapes at bedtime is helpful for many people. Some individuals also need a medication to help them sleep during the crisis around illness. As with pain medicines, people fear addiction to sleep medications far beyond what is warranted, and they end up depriving themselves of something that could help them through the rough spots. If you've never had a drug problem, you're not going to become addicted to a medicine given at bedtime in small doses and on a short-term basis so that you can get a good night's rest. You can stop taking the medicine when the crisis period is over and your normal sleep patterns return, as they usually do. Discuss any sleep problems you're having with your doctor, and share any concerns you might have about taking medication, so that they can be addressed (see Chapter 9 for a more detailed discussion of sleep medications).

Loss of appetite is another common symptom among patients with cancer. It can have many different causes, ranging from the cancer itself to the side effects of treatment to anxiety or depression. Sometimes, the smell or sight of food can trigger a feeling of revulsion after a lengthy course of chemotherapy. Well-meaning family members may become panicky and try to force food on the ill person, which only makes the problem worse. Let your doctor know if you have trouble eating or have lost your appetite. Both psychological approaches and medication can help.

In summary, both physical and psychological symptoms may result in distress that is severe enough to be evaluated and treated. The oncologist is the first line of defense, but some problems require a visit with a professional skilled in recognizing and treating the psychological and psychiatric problems that are common with cancer. Certain life experiences—prior trauma, recent loss of a loved one, or a history of emotional problems—make coping harder and may require referral to a counselor. Anxiety, depression, and confusion are types of distress that respond to treatments targeted to their cause. Pain, nausea and vomiting, fatigue, and loss of appetite often have psychological components. Be sure to avail yourself of help when needed; ask your oncologist for assistance in finding a professional who can address the psychological dimension, or call your local chapter of the American Cancer Society or a nearby cancer center.

THE HUMAN SIDE OF CANCER TREATMENTS

You have probably received much information about the physical side effects of cancer treatment, such as fatigue from radiation or nausea and vomiting from chemotherapy. The psychological side effects usually are not described, however, so they may come as a surprise to you if they happen. We don't usually think of changes in emotions, mental functioning, or mood as side effects to treatment, but it is important to do so, because these reactions are normal and often expected. You may experience none of these, but chances are you'll resonate with at least a few of them at some point. It's better to be prepared so that if you do develop some of the symptoms, you will be better able to deal with them.

When we are highly stressed or in crisis, thoughts, or "mental tapes," repeat themselves in our mind. Following are some thoughts that may run through your head during the course of your treatment.

PSYCHOLOGICAL SIDE EFFECTS OF ALL TREATMENTS

"Are All These Problems Worth the Long-Term Gain?"

When side effects are worst, the trade-off scenario rears its ugly head. Of course, the symptoms are worth tolerating to regain your health and live a longer life. You may have to remind yourself repeatedly of this fact, however, if the going gets rough.

"I'M NOT ME ANYMORE"

Changes in appearance, like losing your hair or looking pale and thin, contribute to a sense of "I'm not me anymore." These physical changes can get you down because they erode that important sense of self-confidence that comes from having your usual appearance. You may hate to look at yourself in the mirror, feel less energetic, and recognize that your body doesn't function the way it did before. Remembering that the symptoms "go with the territory" and will go away when the treatment stops becomes a key to coping.

"I'M BECOMING A HYPOCHONDRIAC"

You may feel that you have no life outside of treatment. This is understandable when you are preoccupied by treatment concerns, watching out for side effects such as fever, and monitoring Mediport care (the Mediport is a catheter placed in a blood vessel under the skin of the chest to draw blood and give chemotherapy without the painful needle sticks in the arms). Dealing with cycle after cycle of chemotherapy begins to make you feel as if the treatment will never end. You may feel that you are obsessed with the function of your body, your illness, and your treatment. This does not mean that you are a hypochondriac. It may seem that way, especially if you haven't paid much attention to your body in the past, when you assumed it would function as it always did. For a while, life must revolve around physical symptoms, medicines, and treatments, but they, too, are temporary.

"AM I A WIMP?"

Major surgery, long hospital stays, and a difficult treatment course can take their toll. Milder symptoms can be difficult as well, for example, repeated low-grade fevers or numbness of fingertips and toes (with chemotherapy). Even patients who experience extremely arduous treatments, such as bone marrow transplantation, often feel that they should be braver or more stoic; people often feel that asking for help is a sign of weakness. You are not a wimp to ask for counseling and support, either on an individual basis or with others going through a similar experience. Ask for information about counseling and support groups and use the resources that are available. If you have more serious problems or feel that you may need medication or a relaxation technique, seek out a counselor or mental health professional who is familiar with the problems caused by cancer.

PSYCHOLOGICAL SIDE EFFECTS OF SURGERY

Surgery is the most common and the oldest treatment for cancer, and it was the only one for a long time. There is still a sense that "cutting it out" is the best treatment. People say, "Well it can't hurt me now that it's out and in a jar." But even if you feel it's the right treatment, it can be frightening to think about being put to sleep and having a surgeon probe around the inside of your body and remove a part of you. Here are some common questions and concerns people have about undergoing surgery.

RELATIONSHIP WITH THE SURGEON

Few other situations call so completely for "placing your life in another person's hands." This is particularly frightening for some people. Finding a surgeon in whom you have trust is a key to dealing with this fear. The next question is, "Who is the best surgeon to do this?" The task is to find out who, in your immediate area, are the experts on your particular type of tumor or operation. A good rule of thumb is to go to someone who performs a particular operation often, not once or twice a year. You want to choose a surgeon who specializes in operating on a specific part of the body and is experienced and technically adept. This often means the surgeon should have additional special training in cancer surgery. Although it's helpful if he or she also has a pleasant bedside manner, that is clearly a secondary consideration in making this choice. If you can have a choice between good hands and good heart, I'd say choose good hands and get psychological support elsewhere. Surgeons may need to maintain a certain emotional distance in order to remove a part of your body and have you live to tell the tale. So it may be asking too much to expect them to be warm and fuzzy at the same time. What is important is that you perceive that the surgeon has a grasp of your particular problem, understands what needs to be done, and is genuinely concerned about your welfare and committed to achieving the best outcome for you.

ANTICIPATION OF SURGERY

As soon as the day and time of the surgery are set, anticipation sets in. You may be one of those people who can put it out of your mind and continue as if this big date did not loom ahead. For others, however, it feels like the agony of countdown until D day.

There has been a 180-degree change in preoperative care from the past, related to the need to reduce costs of care and the role played by managed care in these efforts. You used to come into the hospital the day or at least the night before surgery. You became familiar with the hospital and the nurses and met with the surgeon and anesthesiologist. After a night's sleep and mental preparation, you went to the operating room.

What a change! Today, you will likely come to the hospital to have your laboratory tests and X rays done several days before the surgery. You are told to take no food or drink after midnight the night before your operation and to arrive on time, early in the morning; get into a hospital gown; and go directly to the operating room. I think the current procedure is a negative one from the psychological point of view, especially for those with high anxiety who may need attention to their anxiety and medication to sleep the night before surgery. However, some people like being at home the night before the surgery, in their familiar environment with family. Many patients arise at 4:00 A.M. to drive long distances to arrive at their hospital in time for early-morning surgery.

FEAR OF ANESTHESIA

Like many people, you may be afraid of being put to sleep. This is especially the case if you are the kind of person who needs to be aware of what's going on all the time and in control. Going to sleep evokes the fear of death in some people; the association of sleep and death is common. Fear of anesthesia becomes a kind of phobia and is expressed as "I'm afraid I won't wake up." It is important that the surgeon and anesthesiologist know about your anxiety. You may need preoperative medication to reduce your anxiety when you are being put to sleep.

In the preoperative discussion with you, the anesthesiologist should tell you when, how, and where you will awaken. Knowing the "game plan" reduces the anticipatory distress. A study done many years ago at the Massachusetts General Hospital showed that patients benefited from meeting with their anesthesiologist and having him or her outline exactly what was going to happen in the operating room and afterward in the recovery room. Interestingly, patients who knew what to expect required less pain medication and spent less time in the recovery room than patients who did not have a preop visit with the anesthesiologist. This finding fits in with what we know about the basic human need, mentioned earlier, to "rehearse" frightening events before they occur.

Leaving family and friends while you wait by yourself to go into the operating room can be lonely and stressful. At Memorial Hospital, we have a nun from our chaplaincy service who, every morning, stations herself in the holding area for those waiting to go into the operating rooms. Sister Elaine greets these people and chats with them to reduce their tension. She says a prayer with those who wish her to. Many feel comforted by her kindness and by having a moment to hold a hand and feel the concern of someone after leaving family behind.

FEAR OF THE OPERATION ITSELF

We all like to think of our bodies as remaining intact, without any scars or loss of vital organs or functions. Very few people are so wedded to that idea, however, that they refuse to have needed surgery. When the surgery is going to have a substantial impact, the fear is even greater: loss of an arm or a leg; loss of the voice box; a colostomy, which will require using a bag for bowel function; removal of the bladder, requiring an outlet on the abdominal wall for urine; loss of a breast; or operations that interfere with sexual activity. National organizations have been energetic in reaching out, through their members, to patients who have had a breast removed, a laryngectomy, or a colostomy. These losses of normal body part or function require extensive adaptation to maintain healthy self-esteem and body image.

Fortunately, today more and more procedures are being done with the help of a laparoscope, which is a narrow tube with a camera on the end. This method leads to far smaller incisions, smaller scars, and more rapid recovery. Small incisions are made in two or three places, and cameras and instruments are inserted to excise tissue and simultaneously stop bleeding. This procedure was first used for gall bladder removal, but it is now being used in more complex operations, including those for removing cancers in the lungs and abdomen.

FRIGHTENING MEMORIES OF SURGERY

Because of past experience, the anxiety about an operation can be so great that a person says, "I just can't go through with it." The case of Lou is a good example:

Lou, a fifty-five-year-old married plumber, was told he had esophageal cancer, which might be cured by surgery. He came to the hospital the night before the scheduled operation (back in the days when this was the usual practice) and seemed to be prepared for the surgery. He followed the nurse's instructions and received medication prior to surgery in the morning. He was then wheeled on a cart to the operating room. When he got there, he suddenly panicked and said, "I can't go through with it." The surgery was canceled, and he went home. I was asked to see Lou and evaluate whether he could be helped to go through the procedure at a later time.

We met in my office, and Lou told me that he had managed his life well and had never had any significant psychological problems. However, he had lost his mother when he was eight years old. She had gone to the hospital without telling him she was having a serious operation. He recalled vividly that his father came home and said, "Lou, Mom just died on the operating table." He had grieved for his mother all his life but had managed to keep these painful memories out of his consciousness. However, with the news that he had to have major surgery, the painful memories of his mother's death on the operating table returned vividly. For the week before surgery, Lou had had nightmares, little sleep, and extreme anxiety. He developed a dread that he might die on the operating table as his mother had. We talked over several sessions about the fact that, in reality, the chances of his dying on the operating table were very slim and that his panic represented his long, unresolved grief about his mother. This grief had remained largely controlled until he was confronted with a threat to his own life. He came back to the hospital and was able to go through the operation, which indeed proved curative. Lou is alive and well today.

It's important to remember that long-buried, painful memories, like Lou's, may return to haunt you when you face a crisis of illness; this is an example of posttraumatic stress disorder (PTSD) (see Chapter 11 for a more detailed description of PTSD). Don't be surprised if this happens to you. Usually the problems can be managed, but if they affect your ability to carry out your treatment, you may need to seek help for your distress.

FEAR OF PAIN

Another common fear is that you will be in pain after the surgery. You may have a low pain threshold, or you may have memories of prior surgery that left you in pain and fear of that happening again, which is understandable. You should tell your surgeon about this worry before the operation and ask what pain medicines you can expect to receive. There has been a revolution in postoperative pain management with the widespread use of patient controlled analgesia (PCA) and epidural blocks. The pain medicine, one of the opiates, is placed in an IV bag and is released directly when you, the patient, press a button. It is impossible to administer an overdose. An epidural block places the pain medicine right on the nerves that transmit the pain signals from the operation site as they reach the spinal cord.

These approaches replace the old familiar system in which you waited until the pain got severe and then called the nurse to bring the medication. If the nurse was delayed, you became frightened that the medication wasn't coming and your anxiety increased, thereby setting in motion the cycle of more anxiety and more pain. PCA and epidural blocks are usually in place for a few days following surgery, after which you are switched to a pain medicine that you can take by mouth. It is important to complain whenever the dose of a pain medication is not working for you. Getting the dose right can take careful fine-tuning.

FEAR OF GOING HOME

In these days of managed care, many patients are sent home either on the day of or the day after surgery. (Some health care advocates call these "drive-through" operations.) Some patients are pleased to be able to go home to recover rather than remain in the "antiseptic" hospital environment. However, others fear that they are going home too soon and will be a bother to their family. They also feel more secure under the observation of their doctors and nurses.

Family members may be alarmed that they are expected to provide home care that they feel is out of their league, such as to drain and dress their loved one's wounds. Some people are simply squeamish, while others fear that they will "do it wrong." Whatever the fears and concerns, either on your part or on your family's, speak to your doctor about the possibility of staying in the hospital longer, particularly if you are in pain or feeling weak. The Patients' Bill of Rights ensures that you have the right to request staying in the hospital until a treatment plan is in place (see Chapter 5 on the Patient's Bill of Rights and Chapter 15 on the problems of the family caregiver). If you are concerned that your insurance plan will not cover the cost of a longer stay, ask the hospital social worker to try to straighten this out or to help make arrangements for nursing care at home.

PSYCHOLOGICAL SIDE EFFECTS OF CHEMOTHERAPY

Most people have heard horror stories about chemotherapy. Chemo gets a bad rap. Much of its reputation is due to its early days, when little could be done to make the treatment easier. The nausea and vomiting were particularly bad. If you are carrying the added baggage of having witnessed a parent recovering from chemotherapy in the old days, when nausea and vomiting were so distressing, you may be more upset than others about having chemo. This makes it even more compelling to seek support and encouragement to get through it.

Many people don't realize that there are more than fifty different chemotherapy drugs and an even larger number of combinations of drugs, so that you must ask today: Which drugs? How are they given? What are the benefits and side effects? There is a tendency to assume that all the drugs and combinations are the same, with the same side effects, which is far from true. Some drugs have many side effects that can cause major problems, and others have minimal side effects.

Among the chemotherapy agents for cancers like breast, lung, and other solid tumors, the common side effects are lowered blood counts (making you vulnerable to infections), nausea and vomiting, and loss of hair. Drugs for leukemia and other blood disorders lower blood counts, and there is a wait for normal levels to reappear. Most chemotherapy regimens are given in cycles of treatment, repeated every one to four weeks. This means that a bad week is usually followed by a break, during which you recover. But the cycles can go on for months, and the relentless treatments are almost always accompanied by fatigue, to a greater or lesser degree.

A recent national survey in 1999, conducted by the Oncology Nursing Society and Amgen, Inc. (a pharmaceutical firm), queried people who had been through chemotherapy treatments about the major problems they experienced. Two-thirds of the patients reported a problem before starting the chemotherapy: They felt nervous about what it would be like and what the side effects would be; they felt generally uneasy, not knowing what to expect. Many stated that the time before their first chemotherapy treatment was the worst for them because of their fears. During the chemotherapy, the patients who became depressed were more likely than others to consider stopping treatment. They felt also that others didn't understand what a hard time they were having. They coped by using prayer and getting help from family and others who had also gone through chemotherapy. Some were likely distressed enough that they could have used additional help had it been offered.

It is important that you not respond to fears that you associate with the generic word *chemotherapy*. Most doctors not only explain the drug or drugs to be used, but also give you a fact sheet with information about your particular chemo treatment and the side effects you need to watch out for.

FEAR OF SIDE EFFECTS

Receiving a diagnosis of cancer leads to concerns about the future, but chemotherapy brings out the added fear that the treatment itself has toxic side effects that must be carefully monitored. In fact, the good effect of chemotherapy is the killing of cancer cells anywhere in the body (because the drug goes throughout the body through the bloodstream). This is accomplished at the cost of harming some healthy, normal cells, however, and the cells that grow the fastest are damaged most. Because hair grows rapidly, the follicles are susceptible to the toxic effects of the drugs, leading to thinning of hair or actual baldness. Sometimes there is a loss of body hair. The mucous membrane of the mouth and the lining of the gastrointestinal system can also be affected, so your mouth may become dry, you may get sores in your mouth, or you may have diarrhea. All these effects can be painful; anesthetic mouthwashes and pain medications can help. Numbness and tingling of your fingers and toes can also occur due to the chemotherapy's effects on your nerve endings. This usually disappears some time after the treatment is over.

From a medical point of view, the side effect of most concern is the lowering of your white blood cell count. For this reason, a blood test is done before each chemotherapy treatment to see if the white cell count is high enough to tolerate the next treatment. Today, injections (given at home) can keep the white cell count from dropping and thus prevent infections.*

The red blood cell count can also drop, leading to anemia, which causes fatigue. This side effect can be controlled by transfusion or by a red blood cell stimulating factor called erythropoietin (Epogen or Procrit), which raises the red blood count. The platelet count—platelets are the cells that cause your blood to clot—can also drop during chemotherapy, but platelet transfusions can keep your count closer to the normal range.

We are better able to control nausea and vomiting today than we were even five years ago, and this has changed the experience of chemotherapy enormously for the better. Patients used to tell us they would just look at the calendar and feel nauseated. They might start to vomit on their way to the hospital after their third or fourth treatment. (As described earlier, this is a learned response, like Pavlov's dogs learning to salivate at the sound of a bell.) You may feel some nausea when you think about the treatment or even after your chemo is finished, but this is much less of a problem today than it was in the past. (Chapter 11 describes how some survivors continue to become anxious when they experience or remember a smell or a sight that reminds them of the chemo.)

People nowadays are very interested in natural medicines, without toxic side effects. The idea of enhancing the body's "fighting power" is appealing. When there are viable natural or nontoxic treatments available for a particular medical condition, these, of course, are the first choice. The fact that chemotherapy has toxic effects on normal tissues makes people leery of this potentially life-saving treatment. However, chemotherapy is the most effective treatment we have for many cancers, and it is effective in combination with other treatments for many other types of cancer. Ironically, its very toxicity is the key to its effectiveness in killing off cancer cells. Also, many people are not aware that some of our most effective chemotherapy drugs derive from the active ingredients of medicinal plants. Taxol comes from yew trees; vincristine and vin-

---

*These injections consist of granulocyte-stimulating factor (GSF [Neupogen]), or granulocyte macrophage colony stimutating factor (GM–CSF).

blastine, from periwinkle plants; and Adriamycin from fungi.

The uncertainty and anxiety associated with chemotherapy sometimes become so severe that anxiety itself causes physical symptoms such as dry mouth, a racing heart, and shortness of breath. The anxiety can be as bothersome as the side effects of the toxic drug. The chemotherapy nurses are a superb resource in cancer centers and oncologists' offices. They are experienced in dealing with these problems and can refer you to someone who is able to help.

Mood Swings

Going through the stresses of cancer treatment is enough to make anyone sad, irritable, and frustrated. At times, you may notice that you don't have control of your emotions, and you may cry about minor things. At the other extreme, you may find your mood is a little high and you feel euphoric, without any apparent reason. It is important to know that the cause may be the medications you're taking. For example, both prednisone, which is part of several treatment regimens, and dexamethasone, which is often used to control extreme discomfort from nausea, may affect mood, causing unexplained highs that can be followed by intense lows. This emotional seesaw will pass, and you will return to feeling normal. If the mood swings are severe, ask for help in coping with them; you may even need to take medication to counter them. A persistent low mood could turn into a depression, with the symptoms of sadness, "bad" mood (feeling negative or hopeless), taking no pleasure in things you usually enjoy, and having trouble eating and sleeping. These are signs that you should seek counseling and perhaps receive medication to control these symptoms.

It's important to recognize that these moods are signs of the brain's biochemical reactions to drugs. They do not reflect failure on your part to cope with cancer, nor are they a sign of mental illness. You are fine—it's what the medicines are doing to you.

Irritability

Derek, a thirty-three-year-old man with lung cancer, came in with his wife for a counseling session. His wife said,

"I understand he has cancer and his treatment hasn't been easy. But every little thing sets him off. He's a royal pain in the ass." Derek confirmed that he didn't "feel like myself. I'm 'wired' all the time." Later, I conferred with Derek's oncologist and asked what medication he was taking. As I suspected, he had been receiving a steroid, prednisone, at high doses, which causes a feeling of euphoria at first, but then you may become irritable, moody, and depressed. The reaction can get worse, paradoxically, as the dose is reduced. A few days after the medication was stopped, Derek's usual demeanor returned.

Are you more easily frustrated and annoyed than usual? Is it harder to tolerate frustrations that you usually manage easily? This irritability may be part of your response to the physical and emotional stresses you are experiencing, but it also may be caused by the drugs you are taking. Often the simplest things can help you calm down and feel better, such as soothing music, physical exercise, a warm bath, or relaxation or meditation exercises.

DIFFICULTY CONCENTRATING

While going through chemotherapy, some people complain of having trouble remembering things, reading books and newspapers, and concentrating on their usual work. I recall Sandra, who came to see me because she was so frightened that she simply could not do her work at her law firm. She told me, "I'm losing my mind." She blamed herself for not coping better. She became disconsolate and depressed and considered taking a leave of absence from her highly responsible job. She was taking a high dose of interferon as part of the treatment for melanoma. We were able to control most of the symptoms with an antidepressant medication. When the interferon dose was lowered, her previous level of concentration was restored, her mood returned to normal, and we were able to stop the antidepressant.

We know now that some chemotherapy agents, especially in high doses, may temporarily affect your ability to think clearly, causing memory and concentration problems. Keep in mind that these symptoms usually get better, and you should be back to normal by the time the treatment is over. However, sometimes these difficulties may persist beyond the completion of the treatment; we don't know for how long. Some studies are that finding cognitive changes last as long as two years.

If you find it hard to concentrate during the treatment, try to postpone serious work that requires your full attention for a while. If this side effect persists after the treatment is finished, tell your doctor. Most important, do not blame yourself. In general, problems with concentration are subtle and don't interfere with your normal activities. If you're feeling very distracted or disoriented, check with your doctor about potentially dangerous activities, such as driving. Impaired concentration is usually one of those troublesome side effects that you have to put up with temporarily in exchange for the positive effect of the drug on your tumor.

POOR SLEEP

Although the stress of illness and treatment alone can be sufficient to throw off your sleep-wake cycle, drugs like prednisone also contribute to sleep problems, so trouble sleeping may be a complication of treatment. Try your usual "tricks" to get to sleep, but if you are arising tired and unfit to start your day, ask your doctor for some sleep medication to reset your cycle back to normal.

FATIGUE

While fatigue is a physical symptom, it often feels as though it controls your psychological state as well. During chemotherapy, it can come from low red blood cell counts, causing anemia, or it may be an effect of the treatment on your physical state. Fatigue makes it difficult to get motivated, rouse positive emotions, or undertake physical activities. Some of the high-dose chemotherapy regimens produce profound fatigue, so that for a time, all you can do is simply sit or lie in bed. It may be time to "go with the flow" and get as much rest as you need. Try to remember that the fatigue is a side effect and will go away when the treatment is over. However, it can persist for weeks to months.

PSYCHOLOGICAL SIDE EFFECTS OF RADIATION

Radiation has been used as a treatment for cancer since the early 1900s, soon after its discovery. However, for many years the dose was difficult to control. Only much later on did it become possible to carefully control the dose, so that we could obtain its curative power without intolerable, damaging side effects. For example, cancer of the cervix, larynx, and several other sites can now sometimes be cured by radiation alone. However, most older people remember that when radiation was recommended in earlier days, it meant that the cancer was not curable and it was a palliative treatment (meaning its aim was to delay the growth of the tumor rather than destroy it completely). Almost everybody knows about the radiation damage to people at Hiroshima and Chernobyl, so that the destructive side of radiation is fresh in our memories. Being told that you need radiation treatment for your cancer may arouse these fears: that your cancer cannot be cured or that you might be left with very bad radiation sickness. These are fears based on myths that simply don't apply today; your doctor can explain the reality to you.

FRIGHTENING MEMORIES THAT INCREASE ANXIETY

I recall Doris, who was a retired saleswoman of sixty-nine and a World War II concentration camp survivor. When she went for her first radiation treatment, she panicked when she was isolated in the lead-shielded room and the technician left the room. She was told to lie still until the radiation dose was given. Hearing the click of the switch sent chills through her as she was reminded of her friends who had died in Auschwitz. After a few treatments, she was better able to contain her fears, but because of her understandable anxiety she needed special reassurance each time. This may seem like an extreme example, but radiation can evoke strong fears.

PHOBIAS OF ENCLOSED SPACES

Deborah, a forty-year-old broker who had cancer of the tongue, told me of her fear of being in enclosed spaces. This was a long-existing phobia that didn't usually bother her because she avoided situations that provoked the fear. The radiation treatment required that she be fitted into a mold that was made for her head and shoulders to ensure that she was positioned exactly the same during each treatment. The beam came from a large source lowered from above her. Each time, she required an antianxiety drug before the treatment to control her terror of the machine and the restriction on her motion. A series of frightening thoughts would go through her mind each time she was in the room: The machine might fall on her; the dose might be too high; she might move and the treatment might go to the wrong part of her body. Reassurance, medication, and counseling all helped her to control an old phobia that had caused her little trouble until this new situation required her to face it.

BECOMING FATIGUED

A prominent, almost universal symptom caused by radiation therapy is fatigue, similar to that caused by chemotherapy, although the exact cause of radiation fatigue is not known. The feeling is of lack of energy, inability to carry out your usual tasks, having less interest in your usual activities including sex, and not feeling rested or able to "shake it." Although these symptoms are physical and may come from the radiation, they can also be symptoms of depression, to which you are vulnerable during radiation therapy. Tell your doctor your fatigue is severe and that the cause of it should be sorted out.

The fatigue can linger for weeks after the radiation is completed, so don't be surprised if your energy doesn't rebound quickly at the end of the treatments. High expectations of an immediate return of energy will only make the period more difficult.

BECOMING DEPRESSED

Several people have told me, "You know, Dr. Holland, the reality of my cancer diagnosis didn't sink in until I started the radiation treatments." Coming after the crises of diagnosis and possibly surgery, the daily routine of going for radiation treatment and seeing others who are ill makes you feel the reality more keenly. Don't be surprised if you begin to feel sad as you respond to all that has happened to you. Do ask for help if you need it.

EFFECTS OF RADIATION TO SPECIFIC SITES

Radiation over the chest is apt to affect your swallowing and eating. Loss of appetite and nausea are common, as is a change in the taste of foods, especially if the radiation is over the mouth or throat. Radiation to the chest can affect the esophagus, with discomfort and pain on eating. Diarrhea and loss of appetite, as well as pain, can be side effects of pelvic radiation.

Radiation to the brain causes hair loss, which is often permanent. It may be necessary to get a wig (which is better purchased before the hair loss occurs). You may have a period of poorer concentration while you are receiving radiation to the brain, but your concentration will improve after the treatment ends. In some cases, mild memory problems may persist, such as trouble remembering names. Should this occur, find out if your local hospital or cancer center has a memory-retraining program, which can help you compensate for and cope with this problem. Radiation appears to have remarkably little impact on mood and emotions. However, the steroid drug dexamethasone (Decadron) is often given at the same time, and it can cause mood changes and irritability.

PSYCHOLOGICAL SIDE EFFECTS OF IMMUNOTHERAPY

Increasingly, new therapies are using substances derived from the body that produce an antitumor effect. Immunotherapy is the administration of immune system components such as interferon or interleukin-2 (IL-2) or stimulation of the immune system by vaccines. Interferon is used largely for melanoma, kidney cancer, and some leukemias and lymphomas; IL-2 and monoclonal antibodies and vaccines are being tried with a range of solid tumors. These agents also often have side effects that can make you feel as if you have a bad case of the flu: weakness, fatigue, and at times profound depression, all suggesting an effect on the brain. One person said to me, "I never felt like this in my life. I'm at the end of my rope. I don't understand my despair and hopeless feelings." Some antidepressants, like fluoxetine (Prozac) and paroxetine (Paxil), counter these drug effects well and can reduce the depression when the cancer medication can't be stopped or the dose lowered.

In high doses, these immunotherapies can also cause confusion, especially IL-2, which transiently causes trouble thinking clearly and keeping track of time. You may have a strange feeling that you are seeing something that is not there or misinterpreting something you are seeing, like an illusion. It is good to have a family member around to reassure you and help you keep your thoughts straight. If you experience this side effect, tell your doctor; medications like haloperidol (Haldol) and olanzapine (Zyprexa) are helpful.

PSYCHOLOGICAL SIDE EFFECTS OF BONE MARROW TRANSPLANTATION

Bone marrow transplants (BMTs) are used more frequently today for a wider range of blood disorders and solid tumors than in the past. There are two types: *allogeneic,* in which cells are taken from another person and given to you, and *autologous,* in which your own cells are removed and given back to you at a later time, after high-dose chemotherapy or radiation therapy is completed.

Initially, all BMTs were allogeneic and used exclusively for leukemia. A donor would be found whose bone marrow cells were a "match" for those of the patient. Under anesthesia, the donor had cells removed from the bone marrow (usually the pelvic bones) by multiple needle sticks into the bone. These cells were stored and then given to the patient after receiving chemotherapy and irradiation. Increasingly, autologous transplants are done for types of tumors that don't originate in the blood or bone marrow. Patients' own cells are removed from the bone marrow or, more commonly now, from the blood and returned later after chemotherapy or irradiation treatments are completed. A loss of healthy, normal cells is a side effect of high doses of these cancer treatments, but these cells are replaced by the transfused cells.

The technique being used nowadays is called autologous stem cell transplant (ASCT). The stem cell procedure begins with the patient being given daily injections of a blood cell growth factor (GCSF or GM-CSF), which stimulates the marrow to produce many early progenitor, or stem, cells that eventually develop into red and white cells and platelets. These stem cells are removed from an arm vein by a needle, in a process called leukapheresis. They are then purified, frozen, and stored, to be given to the patient after intensive chemotherapy. ASCT is being used today with the intention of curing leukemia, lymphoma, and Hodgkin's disease, usually when patients have relapsed after primary therapy. It is also being tried in the treatment of several solid tumors, although the success in this case is not clear at the present.

ASCT is a rigorous therapy, often requiring isolation to reduce exposure to possible infection when the white count is low. However, ASCT offers a possible cure to many who have no other option. Side effects of the chemotherapy may involve infections, such as pneumonia; ulcers in the mouth, esophagus, and stomach; loss of hair; and numbness in the hands and feet. Some patients undergoing this treatment receive only high-dose chemotherapy, while others also receive total body irradiation. In either case, great emotional stamina is called for to tolerate the range of problems that can occur over the six to eight weeks of treatment. However, the risks involved are countered by the possibility of long-term benefit and the fact that no other treatment offers similar hope.

Dr. Jerome Groopman wrote in the *New Yorker* about Courtney Stevens who, as a young mother in her early thirties, was facing leukemia. She was told that her only chance to live was to have a bone marrow transplant. She had a clear reason to live—for her children—and a commitment to find the best place to get the best outcome. She went to the pioneering Fred Hutchinson Cancer Research Center in Seattle, where the first bone marrow transplanter, Dr. Donnell Thomas, worked. Groopman calls this treatment "perhaps the worst treatment in all modern medicine—and the best." Courtney did well after the months of punishing treatment, saying confidently and with pride, "What I knew is that I wanted the best shot, the only shot, at a cure, and I've had it."

Groopman calls this treatment the "healing hell" and it is arduous to a degree exceeding most other treatments. No one believes that BMT is an ideal treatment, and oncologists hope that a less disrupting and easier treatment can be found to yield the same results. Until such a treatment comes along, BMT is the best there is to attempt a cure for some tumors. This is clear evidence that we have a long way to go to find an ideal treatment for many cancers.

CLINICAL TRIALS

The best way to prove that a new cancer treatment works and is superior to others is by studying it in clinical trials. Trials are carried out by developing a research protocol in which the therapy is given at a specific dose on a defined schedule to people who have the same stage and type of cancer. Repeated observations are required and specified. The effects on tumor growth can then be determined. It is important that you know something about the why, what, and how of clinical trials, since there are many misunderstandings about them.

First, all clinical trials are under federal regulation, which mandates who is qualified to conduct the studies and requires that each hospital have its own institutional review board (IRB), responsible to the federal oversight agency, to review and monitor every research study being conducted by its staff. The IRB examines the expected benefits of each trial and evaluates the evidence that potential benefits outweigh the risks to the patients. Patients who agree to participate in clinical trials must be informed about all of the risks and benefits, be told about other treatment options available to them, and be told that their care will not be jeopardized if they choose not to participate in the trial. I have been a member of Memorial's IRB for over twenty years. Our IRB is composed of staff physicians and scientists, a patient representative, a chaplain, and two members from the community. All have equal votes.

The federal guidelines for conduct of research on human subjects are derived from the post–World War II Nuremberg trials,
which revealed evidence of terrible abuse of people who were made
the subjects of unethical experiments by Nazi physicians. The resulting outcry after the trials led to the extensive rules we have today to
protect any person who is treated in a clinical trial.

Clinical trials are divided into Phases I, II, and III, each with a
different goal. These phases guide how a new drug or method of
treatment is identified, tested, and finally approved for general use.

Phase I trials are designed to test a new drug or combination of
drugs in humans for the first time and to determine a tolerable dose
of the drug for patients in terms of toxicity. Phase I is the most
experimental phase, and these trials are open only to patients whose
tumors have not responded to the standard treatments available. The
number of patients studied in a Phase I trial is relatively small, rarely
more than twenty. Patients in Phase I trials understand that the drug
has been tried only in animals and that a standard dose has not been
established in humans. Indeed, their informed consent document
states this fact and also that the purpose of the clinical trial is to
determine such a dose. Both patient and doctor hope the drug will
be active, however, and that the patient will be in the first group to
benefit.

Phase II trials constitute the second level of testing of a new drug
or combination of drugs that have undergone testing in a Phase I
trial, during which the safe dose was determined. Phase II trials are
also small, usually composed of about fifteen to forty-five patients.
These patients are studied carefully to determine whether a particular tumor type responds to the drug at the dose and schedule established in the Phase I study. Patients are studied before and after
receiving the treatment to assess the size of the tumor and clinical
benefit. A complete response (CR) means all signs of the tumor have
disappeared, and a partial response (PR) means that the sum of all
the diameters of all the tumors has decreased by half. Phase II trials
often test a new drug or combination of drugs in several different
types of tumors. For example, gemcitabine (Gemzar) was first shown
to be effective in pancreatic cancer. It was tested in other Phase II
trials and found valuable in the treatment of other tumors as well.

Patients who choose to participate in Phase II trials understand that standard, available treatments may not be effective against their tumors and that, while there is no assurance of benefit as a result of the new treatment, there is hope that the drug will be effective for them.

Phase III trials study drugs that have proved to be effective treatments in Phase II trials and that appear to be as good as or better than standard treatments for a particular tumor. A Phase III trial is termed a randomized controlled trial. Patients are assigned to either the standard treatment or the new one by a chance mechanism, hence the term randomized.

Patients participate knowing that they will receive either the best standard treatment or the experimental one, which may be better. They cannot choose, however. No placebo or sugar pill treatments are used; the best standard treatment is compared with the new one. Several hundred patients are recruited for Phase III studies, which are often conducted by the large cooperative clinical trials groups directed by the National Cancer Institute. Patients are matched as nearly as possible for any other factor that might affect response or survival, like level of physical performance, age, menopausal status, or prior treatment. The size of the study groups for Treatment A and Treatment B is determined by statisticians on the basis of the size of any expected difference. If the investigators think a new treatment would be of interest only if it could double the response rate, or double the survival rate, they will take fewer patients than if they are willing to settle for a treatment that will improve these parameters by only 25 percent. The outcome of this large study is then presented to the Food and Drug Administration. If the new treatment turns out to be more effective than the standard one, the results are announced to doctors, who then can use it as first-line therapy.

To be sure that the two groups are nearly identical and that there is no bias in choosing which patients go into either group, participants must agree to be assigned randomly to receive either the experimental treatment or the standard treatment. Which group you go into is determined by a centralized computer that your doctor doesn't control. The reason for this randomization is the notion that doctors or patients might be biased if they were allowed to select the treatment the patient will get. It is critical that the determination of groups be unbiased. This is sometimes a sticking point for patients, and may be for doctors, but it is the only way to determine when a new treatment is truly better. It is crucial to remember that you will receive either the current best treatment for a tumor or one that may be even better. No investigator plans to study a treatment regimen that he or she thinks is less effective than the standard.

As difficult as these trials seem, they are essential for improving the treatment of cancer, which stills falls far short of where everyone wants it to be. When you take part in a clinical trial, you are carefully monitored, your treatment options are fully explained, you get either the best treatment known or possibly a better one, and you contribute to improving treatment of future cancer patients.

Some people are afraid of clinical trials because they think they will be treated less well: "I'll just be a guinea pig." This is far from true since much preparation and review goes into the protocol plan, watching for side effects, and observing tumor response. In a study of children treated in clinical trials compared with those who were not, survival was better among the children treated in trials.

In many trials today, investigators also monitor the functioning of patients in the different areas of their lives, that is, the physical, psychological, social, work, and sexual domains. These data constitute what is called "health-related quality of life," which yields scores that are then used to measure not only length of survival, but also the quality of that survival.

Others who are ill become upset when a particular clinical trial isn't available to them because their medical status doesn't exactly fit the criteria set out in the protocol. I have seen people who were bitterly disappointed at not being able to take a new experimental treatment, especially people for whom standard treatment has failed and who are seeking treatment on Phase I and II protocols. It is hard to balance the demands of doing good science that gives solid answers versus the human needs of people who are seriously ill. At times, in exceptional situations, an IRB will give permission for a "compassionate exception," so that a doctor can treat someone who does not meet the criteria for participation in the trial.

There are added psychological strains on both the physician, who is at the same time a clinical investigator and a personal physician, and the patients, who are very aware of how much is riding on the outcome of the experimental treatment for themselves and others. The doctor and patient become partners not only in treatment, but in research. I'm always amazed at the altruism of the many people who say, "Maybe it won't help me, but I'm glad to be helping to find a better treatment for patients with cancer who will come after me."

Without clinical trials, better treatments for cancer cannot be found. The human side of clinical research is as important as the human side of clinical care. Clinical trials require a high level of trust between the doctor and the patient and knowledge that improvement is possible, providing the basis for hope.

In summary, the main treatments for cancer—surgery, radiation, chemotherapy, and immunotherapy—have some common physical side effects and some common psychological side effects. Anxiety or depressed feelings sometimes arise from dealing with illness, but also arise from the treatments themselves. Thanks to psychological support through family, friends, clergy, and group and individual therapy, there are ways to help you tolerate the treatments. Medications to control sleeplessness, anxiety, mood swings, and poor concentration are available. Such drugs are not addictive when taken under supervision and can bring great relief from troublesome symptoms. Self-managed methods of relaxation and meditation are also effective. Use what suits you and your personality best. The important thing is: Don't suffer in silence. There *is* help available if you ask for it. If participation in a clinical trial is offered to you as a possible treatment option, be sure to obtain full information by reading the materials given to you and talking with the physician. Becoming a partner in a clinical investigation is a helpful way of coping for many people. You can get a listing and description of all available clinical trials for different tumors by either phoning the information line (1-800-4-CANCER) or visiting the website of the National Cancer Institute (see Resources).

THE HUMAN SIDE OF SPECIFIC CANCERS

Losing a breast was very hard, but I had a lot of support and I've gotten through it. Now that I'm feeling back to my old self, I'm worried about my daughter and granddaughters getting cancer and having to go through what I did. It keeps me up at night.

—Olivia, a fifty-eight-year-old breast cancer survivor

I hate this bag, even though I can't live without it. I know other people have adjusted to having one, but some days I feel like I never will.

—Ross, who recently had a colostomy after treatment of colon cancer

I've always been a very private person, especially about my body, and now all these doctors keep examining me and I feel embarrassed and exposed.

—Ellen, a woman with endometrial cancer

*I*f you have experienced cancer, or a family member has, you must have questions about the human side of that particular cancer. The earlier chapters of this book have focused on the universals of coping with distress, worry, and fears for the future. But each cancer presents its own problems and treatment. This chapter deals with those specifics. (The Resources section outlines the national organizations that deal with cancer in general and those that provide information about specific tumors.)

BREAST CANCER

How do you cope with cancer in the breast, which gets at the very heart of what we as women hold dear, our femininity? Virtually every treatment for breast cancer is an assault on femininity: Surgery removes a part or all of the breast; chemotherapy can cause your hair to fall out and a premature menopause with cold and hot flashes, mood swings, irritability, and sexual problems including less desire and vaginal dryness; radiation therapy causes fatigue. And the ultimate stressful treatment today, high-dose chemotherapy and bone marrow transplant, was described by Dr. Jerome Groopman as "healing hell" (see Chapter 7).

What helps in coping with these problems?

1. Before treatment, ask questions about what you can expect. It's better to be prepared so that you aren't taken off guard. Maintaining a healthy self-image is central. Losing part or all of a breast, although traumatic, is not as bad as losing your life. Your hair will grow back, the menopausal symptoms will go away, fatigue will finally diminish, sexual counselors can help with your sex problems, and your doctor can recommend lubricants for vaginal dryness.

2. Your anxiety is probably highest in that period after receiving the diagnosis, when you are deciding about treatment. Research shows that high anxiety actually makes it harder to process information, just at the time you most need your faculties about you. You may be unable to make a decision because anxiety is so high. If that is the case, you should see a counselor, and you may need a prescription for an antianxiety medication from your doctor.

3. Talk with women who have been through the treatment. Reach to Recovery, the American Cancer Society program that provides assistance to women in the hospital after breast surgery, is a built-in plus. Women do well sharing their problems with other women. You will find breast cancer support groups in most cities today. They work for many women.

4. Look Good, Feel Better is a national program cosponsored by cancer centers and cosmetologists in most cities. You can have a "makeover," in which you try on makeup to hide pale or blemished skin; learn ways to wear scarves, turbans, or hats in fashionable ways to hide baldness; and get suggestions for choosing the right wig. Call your local chapter of the American Cancer Society.

5. Be open with others about your diagnosis and treatment unless there is a compelling reason to conceal it. Tell a prospective sexual partner about your breast cancer sooner rather than later. A man who can't tolerate the information isn't one you want to consider seriously anyway.

6. If you have a partner, it's best to involve him (or her, in lesbian couples) in the visits to the doctor from Day 1. Sharing the experience leads to talking about it together, and the partner should be a part of each step from diagnosis through the operation to changing the dressings after surgery. If you have no partner, it helps a great deal to have a friend who's there for you at times like this.

7. Involving your partner makes the return to sexual activity much more natural. The standoff that can occur—with the partner thinking, "I don't want

to hurt her," and the woman with breast cancer feeling, "I'm not desirable anymore"—is diminished. Seek a sex counselor if things don't go well, if possible one who is experienced in the sexual problems related to cancer. Sometimes, the problem is more emotional than physical (for example, fear of painful intercourse, anxiety, or depressed feelings) and seeing a counselor will help.

8. If you are worried about your daughter's or sister's risk of breast cancer because of your diagnosis, suggest she go to a genetic counseling program for breast cancer, where a careful family history will be taken to determine her actual level of risk. She will be given a plan for monitoring herself to ensure early diagnosis: instructions on how to do monthly breast self-examinations and advice on getting regular breast examinations and mammograms. Support groups are helpful for women who realize they are at risk by virtue of their family history. Some women's level of distress is as high as that in women who are survivors of breast cancer. Knowing your daughter or sister is being monitored may relieve some of your anxiety as well.

Susan's experience tells us something about the human side of breast cancer:

A single woman of thirty-eight, Susan was focused on a highly successful business career. Although she was in a new relationship, she felt that marriage and children could be safely delayed and that there was no reason to worry too much about her biological clock. However, on showering one day she felt an alarming, hard lump in her right breast. A mammogram showed, to her amazement, a 3-cm shadow in her right breast. Accustomed to being able to take steps to fix any problem that occurred, she was thrown off guard by a problem that wasn't so easily fixed. Owing to the size and apparently aggressive nature of the tumor, two surgeons recommended a mastectomy followed by adjuvant chemotherapy instead of a lumpectomy and radiation. She was devastated by her concerns: How will I look? Whom should I tell? What should I say? How shall I tell my new friend, and possible partner, who is clearly interested in me, about having breast cancer? Do I tell him now or do I wait until he sees the mastectomy scar and tell him then? How do I tolerate losing my hair? What will the chemotherapy do to my ovaries? Will it affect my ability to have children?

Susan struggled with these worries, but she recognized that she had to make a decision for her future life and health; she couldn't wish the problem away. She talked with other women who had been through the same situation, women she knew and friends of friends, who generously shared their own experience. She decided to have a mastectomy with an immediate reconstruction at the time of the mastectomy. This course worked out well. Before starting chemotherapy, Susan bought a wig that was a true match to her own hair. As her hair began to fall out, she was distressed, but she wore her wig and was surprised to discover that few people noticed the difference. She was able to work during the course of the chemotherapy. She developed hot flashes and noticed she was more easily upset and irritable, but these reactions diminished as the chemotherapy was completed.

Within a year, Susan's life was back on track, and she began to feel that it was possible to have a normal life. She had decided to tell her friend before the surgery, and he supported her through the treatments. As he said, "I'm interested in you, not your breast." She realized that if she couldn't have her own child, alternatives were open to her to have a child through a surrogate mother or adoption. Susan's future looked bright when I saw her two years later, and she was happily married.

In rare cases, breast cancer may occur in men. If you are one of those men, you may have encountered the stigma of people reacting strangely or in disbelief to your having "a woman's disease." There is much less support available for men with breast cancer, so you may wish to get individual counseling.

GYNECOLOGIC CANCER

The human side of gynecologic tumors involves many of the same issues encountered with the diagnosis of breast cancer. They are outlined below, along with suggestions for coping with them.

1. *A sense of loneliness.* There is a stigma associated with gynecologic cancer. You may feel embarrassed to tell anyone except your family and closest friends. You may feel uncomfortable having people speculate about your sexual issues after having gynecologic cancer. The isolation also makes it harder to share your worries with others about the threat that cancer poses to your life.

Talking with women who have had the same tumor is helpful. Support groups are available in most places today. Getting connected to an organization in your community for people with your particular cancer can make all the difference. You realize you aren't alone. You learn practical ways of coping. For example, several organizations are devoted to ovarian and cervical cancer (see Resources at the end of the book).

2. *Sexual problems.* Your unacknowledged fear about a diagnosis of gynecologic cancer is "what will happen to my sex life?" It's a key question, and yet you may hesitate to ask the doctor about it. The doctor doesn't discuss it, and the fear grows, as you go through treatment.

Sarah Auchincloss, a psychiatrist in my group, specializes in treating sexual problems associated with cancer (see Chapter 9 for a discussion of sexual counseling). She points out that every woman has a sex life that is threatened by gynecologic cancer. Women who have an active sex life fear treatment will end it. Women who don't have an active sex life feear they may never have one. All women are concerned about attractiveness, desirability, and keeping relationships in which sex has been a part. Fear about losing relationships causes great anxiety.

Auchincloss makes a second point. All women with gynecologic cancer can keep a partner sexually happy, despite physical changes caused by illness. Most women in this situation are more concerned about keeping their partner satisfied than about their own gratification. It is good to remember that even if desire is reduced or absent, or if it isn't possible to have sex in your accustomed way, it's still possible to be a good lover. Touching, closeness, and caressing are all important, and oral or manual stimulation can lead to orgasms if vaginal intercourse is painful or impossible (by virtue of fatigue or narrowing or shortening of the vagina). People's sex lives evolve over time as they make adaptations in their sexual practices to age, illness, or disabilities. It's important that you don't assume that if sex can't be like it used to be, you must give it up altogether. If you avoid sex and don't talk about it, you adopt the attitude of "there's an elephant in the room, but we won't mention it." This approach puts more strain on the relationship at a time when closeness means everything.

Auchincloss's third point is that sexual problems, while common after cancer treatments, are treatable. A return to sex should occur when desire returns and healing has occurred. Ask your doctor about timing. If your vagina is shortened by scarring or fibrosis from radiation treatment, you will find lubricants helpful; should you want to have intercourse, you can experiment to find a comfortable position. If pain occurs, your doctor or a sex counselor can suggest exercises and ways to reduce anxiety. Regular vaginal dilatations using vaginal dilators with a lubricant may be recommended to avoid narrowing. Remember that sexual problems create emotional problems, and vice versa. You cannot separate these physical problems from their emotional components. A counselor should be able to assess both.

3. *Menopausal problems.* Premature menopause develops as a result of surgery that removes the ovaries, and also from radiation and chemotherapy, which affect ovarian function. Hot flashes, mood swings, irritability, and depressed mood go along with the abrupt hormonal changes that accompany these treatments. If not contraindicated, estrogen replacement will reduce these problems. Also, a medication like sertraline (Zoloft) is effective in reducing severe hot flashes. Mood changes may need to be treated by antidepressants. Discuss these problems with your doctor; if appropriate, the doctor will refer you to a counselor.

4. *Infertility.* Ovarian tumors may require treatments that result in infertility. The ovaries are affected by the extent of the surgical procedure and by radiation and chemotherapy. It is possible that in the future, ovaries, or at least their ova, can be stored by freezing (as sperm currently are), but these procedures are not yet available. Surrogate mothers are increasingly being used, and adoption is an option that should be considered. It can be an enormous emotional challenge to deal with the loss of your ability to have your own biological child; counseling may be crucial to your efforts. Everyone recognizes what a significant loss this is for many young women. Fortunately, today, support groups are available for women with infertility problems (see Resources).

GENITOURINARY CANCERS

PROSTATE CANCER

If you have had prostate cancer, you may have had surgery (prostatectomy), radiation, chemotherapy, or hormonal treatment. Surgery can cause incontinence, which is difficult to cope with. Erectile dysfunction (impotence) is another common side effect of surgery, as well as of radiation and hormonal therapy. Treatment with estrogen to lower testosterone levels leads to troublesome feminizing characteristics, such as breast enlargement, redistribution of fat tissues, and mood swings.

You may find it hard to let your partner know how distressed you are about these changes. It's a bind that raises important issues for men in our society. Men ought to feel free to connect with their feelings and express them, especially to those they love. But to the contrary, American society still discourages men from talking about their own feelings and emotional problems. Not surprisingly, you may feel isolated in dealing with your feelings and in sharing what you know is sensitive and difficult.

What helps in coping? First, be open to looking at yourself and to exploring your own sense of self. You may find yourself depressed (more than just sad) a lot of the time during treatment. If you have a partner, he or she is likely to be sad, too. We found women whose partners had prostate cancer had as much distress as their spouses, but they wouldn't let their partners know it.

Is the need for repeated prostate specific antigen (PSA) tests something that makes you worry and feel pessimistic about the future? The real worry is what's going to happen if a PSA test shows that you have a tumor or that the tumor is growing. If you have these concerns, consider counseling for yourself and/or your partner. Talking with other men is another way of coping; you can do this through groups like Man to Man and Us Too in most cities. It's helpful to hear other men speak directly about their experiences because they are likely to be similar to yours.

How do you cope with impotence? Most surgeons today are

skilled at sparing the pelvic nerves that control erection. Still, impotence often results from prostate surgery, and partial or complete impotence remains a common side effect of radiation, as well as of hormonal therapy through the lowering of the testosterone level. Several types of penile implants are available today, requiring only a minor surgical procedure. Injections of agents that cause constriction of blood vessels in the penis can produce an erection. When nerve damage results from prostate surgery, in general, stimulants such as sildenofil (Viagra) are not generally highly effective. Your doctor can refer you to one of the many urologists who specialize in this area today.

It is important to remember that you can still be a good lover by remaining affectionate and loving. Avoiding sex completely is not a solution. Touching, caressing, and producing an orgasm by oral or manual stimulation keeps the meaningful sexual relationship intact. You and your partner can adapt so that your sex life continues despite illness. Sexual counseling is helpful for improving communication, reducing anxiety or depression, and suggesting sexual techniques.

BLADDER CANCER

Bladder cancer occurs in older women and men. You may have been through repeated cystoscopies and treatment of the bladder wall. The human side requires coping with these repeated procedures and the fear that a biopsy will find that the cancer has spread. If it invades the bladder wall, a cystectomy may be recommended to remove the bladder. This major procedure may include the construction of a false bladder called Koch's pouch to collect urine from the ureters. You can cope best with having the pouch by getting detailed instructions about its management and by talking with others who have been through the procedure.

This tumor of older years comes on when other losses are occurring in your life. Depression is a risk, and you should seek counseling through your doctor if you experience a significant level of distress.

Increasing numbers of organizations are devoted to education about urological cancers and advocacy for research (see Resources).

TESTICULAR CANCER

This tumor of young men has a difficult human side: coping with cancer at a young age and coping with the treatment's side effects. You have to face having a testicle removed by surgery and chemotherapy treatment for the tumor at a time in your life when you want to look and feel "normal." Nowadays, prostheses are available so that the scrotum looks normal and you can feel confident about seeking and maintaining an intimate relationship. However, chemotherapy frequently causes infertility, because it kills sperm cells in the remaining testicle. The good news is that now you can bank sperm before beginning treatment so that your sperm cells will be available later if you want to father a child. Also, testicular surgery removes lymph nodes near the pelvic nerves in the abdomen, causing the ejaculate to be small in amount or absent; however, the surgery has no effect on erection. It helps to be well informed up front about these matters, to bank sperm, and to join a support group for young adults with cancer, who face problems similar to yours (see Resources). If you have serious distress or concerns, seek individual psychotherapy.

GASTROINTESTINAL (GI) CANCER

If you have a tumor of the GI tract, you know the troublesome human side of coping with loss of appetite and enjoyment of food, nausea, constipation, diarrhea, or pain with eating. Tumors of the esophagus, stomach, colon or rectum, pancreas, and liver all may cause these problems, as do their treatments.

Treatment is apt to involve surgery, chemotherapy, and possibly radiation. The effects of surgery will depend on how extensive the resection to remove the tumor is. You can expect to resume your full activities; remember that President Ronald Reagan continued to work in the Oval Office after having a colon cancer removed.

A colostomy (pertaining to the colon) or ileostomy (pertaining to the small bowel) is necessary when the ends of the bowel cannot be reconnected. Both of these surgeries take a great human toll because of having to adjust to a bag on the abdomen. You have to deal with fears of bad odors, unsightliness, and the feeling of being unacceptable to a sexual partner, as John's story illustrates:

> John, a fifty-year-old, fastidious engineer, was diagnosed with colon cancer. The surgeon indicated that he might have to do a wide resection to remove all the tumor, and a permanent colostomy might be necessary. John reluctantly signed his consent but was devastated when he awakened from the surgery with an ostomy opening in his abdomen. He became depressed and refused to learn how to care for the bag. He felt he would be too humiliated to ever try to have sexual relations with his wife with "that thing between us." Good counseling came from the ostomy nurse, an "ostomate" herself, who gave him the courage to cover the ostomy and try sex again. Over several months, he became more confident. He later became an active volunteer to help others who had his fears, concerns, and dread.

The United Ostomy Association, an umbrella organization for people with an ileostomy or colostomy, can put you in contact with your local chapter (see Resources).

When you cope with some GI tumors, like pancreas and liver cancer, you must deal with reading repeatedly about the dire statistics associated with those diseases. You have to keep in mind that you aren't a statistic, you are one person, and that these tumor types are best looked at as a kind of chronic illness. You may not be able to look to a cure, but the goal is that present treatments will keep the cancer controlled until better, more curative treatments are available. My oncologist husband, who sees things in the "glass is three-quarters full" mode, calls such tumors "precurable," since he is certain new, targeted treatments are coming. He says there are no noncurable tumors, only precurable ones.

Colon cancer carries an extra psychological burden: the concern for what your diagnosis may mean for your children and siblings. There has been much progress in identifying the gene for some colon cancers that seem to run in families. Your oncologist should be able to refer you and your family to a center that can study your family history, and a genetic counselor can recommend the follow-up that other family members should have. Regular colonoscopies may be recommended to detect polyps (growths that may develop into cancer) and any signs of early cancer, if the risk is thought to be high enough to warrant surveillance.

LUNG CANCER

The human side of lung cancer presents a dual burden: the burden of the illness itself, and the sense that others are blaming you for having been a smoker. However, not everyone who gets lung cancer was a smoker; about 10 percent of people who develop lung cancer never smoked in their life. Whether or not you smoked, the assumption of guilt by others increases the sense of isolation. This is why psychosocial support is so important for you if you have lung cancer. A woman who had lung cancer urged me to start a support group for lung cancer patients. At that time, no such group existed for our patients. She put it so well: "Would you believe I sit in the waiting room and *wish* that I had breast cancer—there is so much more support for them." Another woman told me that when she came to the support group, it was the first time she had spoken with any other person who had lung cancer. No one else understands quite like another who is going through the same experience (see Chapter 9 for a discussion of group support).

To handle the human side of lung cancer, remember the following:

1. The American Lung Cancer Association for Support and Education (ALCASE) is the national association for lung cancer patients; its telephone number is 1-800-298-2436. This organization has a wealth of information about support groups and where they're located. It also has a "buddy" system and will put you in touch with someone in your area (see Resources).

2. Get maximal support from your oncology team. The oncology nurse is often the linchpin in terms of being there for you and listening to your problems.

3. If you are having a lot of anxiety or if you are getting depressed, ask the oncology team for a referral for extra psychological help.

4. If you are a smoker, support is available to help you quit (see Chapter 12).

HEAD AND NECK CANCER

If your tumor is of the face, mouth, or throat, the human side of coping is especially difficult. It is a great burden if the tumor or the treatment changes your appearance, your eyes, or your voice. Yet many such patients have managed well with the aid of plastic surgery, prostheses inside the mouth to help in chewing and swallowing, and use of an artificial speech method that entails placing a vibrator to the throat that amplifies sounds and creates understandable speech. One courageous survivor, Jay Lemaster, spoke at a recent cancer conference using his assisted speech device, which has been his method of communication for the past five years, since his voice box was removed. He joked about sounding like a robot, but he spoke to 250 cancer survivors, giving hope to everyone present. There is no doubt that improvements in the technology of assisted speech are coming.

What will help you cope with a tumor in one of these areas?

1. Be sure to get sufficient support from your oncology team, and use the oncology nurse as your closest contact with the team. Through this team, resources are readily accessible, such as support group meetings and the laryngectomy organiza-

tion. The national organization Support for People with Oral and Head and Neck Cancer (SPOHNC) will put you in touch with psychological services (see Resources).

2. Don't become a recluse because of shyness about the way you look or speak following treatment. Keep up your relationships with people who you know will not feel differently about you because of the physical changes. As you gain confidence, you can return to work and resume your social activities.

3. Depression is often a complicating problem. Do seek consultation and treatment for it.

HEMATOLOGIC MALIGNANCIES

This category includes a range of disorders of the blood, including Hodgkin's disease, leukemia, lymphoma, and multiple myeloma. If you have one of these disorders of the blood and lymph glands, you know that the fields of hematology and oncology have made big strides in their treatment. However, the treatments are grueling because they require cycles of intensive chemotherapy and sometimes high-dose chemotherapy and blood or marrow transplants.

Getting through the treatments is difficult, but with a goal of cure, the side effects become more tolerable. You should anticipate losing your hair and get a wig early. Be prepared for some nausea and perhaps vomiting. You may find, later, that every time you encounter a reminder of the treatment, like being in the treatment room or even smelling alcohol, you may get nauseated again as a conditioned response (see Chapters 6 and 9 for more details, including ways to relieve these symptoms).

Gordon, a young Hodgkin's disease survivor, had been successfully treated in his teens. The disease recurred, however, and this time he underwent a stem cell transplant. He remembered his chemotherapy from ten years earlier, when there was poor control of nausea and vomiting, and dreaded facing it a second time. When he came into the hospital for the chemotherapy, before receiving the stem cells he asked that the bags of chemotherapy be covered so he could pretend he was getting something like Perrier. This helped to hold those old associations at bay. After he recovered, he described seeing someone in the supermarket one day and suddenly becoming anxious and nauseated. It was only then that he recognized the person as the nurse who had given him the chemotherapy in the hospital many months earlier. He realized why it was happening, took some deep breaths, and was able to relax.

You may be surprised by having long periods of fatigue after treatment. If you expect your normal energy to return too soon, you may think, "Am I doing something wrong?" No, you aren't. Be patient about getting back to your former activity level. It may take some time.

Anxiety and depressed mood are common during chemotherapy so don't be alarmed should they occur, especially if you are undergoing high-dose chemotherapy with a stem cell transplant. Ask for a counselor in the hospital or in the clinic when you come back for visits (see Chapter 7). Meditation, relaxation exercises, and medication may help.

After the treatment is over, you may develop symptoms of posttraumatic stress disorder (PTSD), such as restlessness, becoming easily startled, and being unable to concentrate or enjoy life. This reaction usually diminishes over a few months, but if it persists you need to seek evaluation and treatment, likely with medication and psychotherapy. (PTSD can develop after a highly stressful or traumatic event. Chapter 11 discusses PTSD among cancer survivors in greater detail.)

MELANOMA AND SARCOMA

MELANOMA

If you have a malignant melanoma, you probably are young, look healthy, and find that nobody can believe you are ill. The incision left after removing the tumor looks innocuous enough, but you are living with with the uncertainty that the cancer might come back, requiring repeated surgery and immunotherapy. You may find it hard to talk with others about your illness; friends may not want to hear about it and they won't understand. So you feel isolated from others. One young woman told me, "I feel like I have two lives. I look okay and go out on dates, but I feel deceitful, as if I am living a lie. I make up wild stories about how I got my scars, like being in a car accident or on a motorcycle. It's hard living one life of cancer and another of 'pretend health.'"

Because you are unlikely to know anyone else with the same tumor, support groups are valuable. You can express your fears with others who do understand and share your concerns about how hard it is to form a serious relationship. Another plus is that there's much discussion in the groups of telling or not telling others about the illness.

SARCOMA

Sarcomas are tumors that arise in the muscle and bone; they can develop anywhere in the body. Like melanomas, sarcomas also occur among young, healthy-looking people, so the diagnosis is usually a great shock to you and your loved ones. It is hard to find a support group for people who have sarcoma because it is so uncommon. Treatment of osteosarcoma may require amputation. The loss of a limb and the rehabilitation process make this a difficult psychological adjustment. And with the loss comes the stigma of being different and the feeling that "everybody is staring at me," which is particularly hard for adolescents and young adults, who are more prone to this type of cancer. Of course a basic worry is that you might not be able to live a normal life anymore or take part in your favorite activities. Media coverage of Ted Kennedy Jr.'s adjustment to the amputation of a leg due to a sarcoma of the bone, with photos of him skiing while wearing a prosthesis, did much to dispel these fears.

You may have to search out a support group for people with sarcoma who are about your own age, since problems vary by age. Trying to find the right support group is best pursued by contacting the American Cancer Society (see Resources).

BRAIN TUMORS

The human side of illness is particularly poignant with reference to brain tumors. First, there is the fright and dread you feel when you're told that you have a brain tumor. How can you begin to adjust to such painful news? The diagnosis is a threat to your life, and also a threat to your "thinking." After all, our head is where we live. The treatment is the next forbidding prospect you face, and it is apt to be surgery, from which you will recover quickly. If radiation follows, this will be a more trying time since it usually continues over several weeks and results in hair loss. Fortunately, it usually causes few side effects related to thinking. If you do have trouble, you can meet with a neuropsychologist to learn how to use special tricks to improve your memory and other skills. You may also have taken steroids (for example, Decadron) during the period of surgery and radiation therapy. This drug can cause mood changes, depression, and weakness (see Chapter 7).

The human fallout will be much easier to deal with if you find support services for yourself and your family. Talking with others about coping with a brain tumor can be mighty helpful. However, you may be the type of person who is more comfortable speaking alone with a therapist about the burdens you are carrying from this illness and how best to cope.

You may need medication to control distressing symptoms. Your neurologist can suggest a psychiatrist who provides psychological services for patients with brain tumors. Special services are available in many locations across the country. You can contact your local

American Cancer Society, the Brain Tumor Society, or the National Brain Tumor Foundation (see Resources).

In summary, in coping with the human side of illness, the first line of support is your family and your oncology team. In addition, many organizations have been formed to help you find information and support to deal with specific tumors. The place to start is with the national organizations, like the National Cancer Institute (1-800-4-CANCER) and the American Cancer Society (1-800-ACS-2345). The Resources section of this book lists these organizations along with organizations whose goals are specific to a particular type of cancer. These societies, foundations, and groups are also able to refer you to a psychological counselor who is familiar with your illness.

ALL MEDICINE DOESN'T COME IN A BOTTLE: PSYCHOLOGICAL TREATMENTS

My life was pretty messed up when I got cancer. After the treatment was over, I vowed I'd take advantage of this new chance to straighten some things out. I started psychotherapy to help with a career I had always wanted, but had given up. I'd keep shooting myself in the foot and couldn't figure out why. Psychotherapy got me clear about it, and I got some insight on how I was living out my life. Truth is I wouldn't have done this if I hadn't gotten a wake-up call from cancer.

—Bill, a leukemia survivor

I was so afraid of the cancer treatment. I couldn't make up my mind to have a bone marrow transplant, which they said was my one chance for a cure. I asked the doctor for help, and a counselor took me, mentally, step by step, through what was coming up, and gave me support through the first treatments. It got me through it. I might have refused the treatment otherwise and missed my chance for a cure.

—Jan, a Hodgkin's disease survivor

I heard about meditation and mind-body tricks to help you stay calm when you're nervous. I learned to practice meditation and relaxation, and they got me through my fears of surgery and the pain after it. Now,

I have this in my own bag of tricks to use when I'm going to the dentist or through bad stress.

> —Karen, a survivor of ovarian cancer

At first, groups turned me off. I didn't like the idea of having to listen to other people's symptoms. If they were sicker than I, that would start me worrying about myself; if they were not as sick, that would make me jealous. But it actually turned out that we were all in the same leaky boat. We really could understand what each other felt. They became like friends to me, and I could count on them to listen to me and ease my worries. There was a camaraderie that I'd never felt before, and it carried me through some terrible days.

> —David, a member of a lung cancer group

I hate medicines of all kinds. I don't even take aspirin for a headache. I was afraid to take anything to sleep, even though I was staying awake all night worrying about the surgery. I would get up too tired and depressed to face a new day. My doctor suggested that I see the psychiatrist who works with him. After a couple of visits, I came to see that taking something would be better than the way things were for me. So I willingly took a mild sedative to get some sleep at night and that made it a little easier to do what I had to do during the day. The best part is that I got through my surgery okay.

> —Alex, after colon cancer surgery

You may be an extraordinarily good coper or you may find you have trouble just making it through some days. Either way, coping with cancer taxes your ability to the maximum. I believe you can benefit from knowing about the types of psychological help that are available and trying those that appeal to you. The approaches outlined were culled from techniques and therapies in general use; they are included because they have been found effective with people who have cancer. I discuss the various available treatments: individual and group counseling, cognitive-behavioral techniques (ways of viewing illness that help), relaxation, meditation, prayer and spiritual practices, art and music therapies, creative writing, and medications for problems not adequately relieved by other methods.

COUNSELING

Feeling sad and worried is normal at times during cancer treatment, no matter how good a coper you were before the illness. Indeed, the word *cancer* itself evokes these feelings because of its meaning and implications. You may be someone who copes so well that, with the help of your family and friends, you manage the crises of illness well. On the other hand, you may be a person who finds it hard to cope some days. In this case, you can find help by talking with a counselor or by sharing your concerns and feelings with others who are going through the same experience you are. If you are having serious problems, like anxiety or depression, you may benefit from a medication that can be prescribed by your oncologist or a psychiatrist who works with patients who have cancer. Keep in mind that these problems "go with the territory" of cancer; they are normal reactions to the illness. They are not a sign of a psychiatric illness or of personal weakness. Getting help makes good sense.

If you have had emotional problems in the past or lost someone dear to you to cancer, you may have more trouble coping. It is tempting to try to be strong and bear it alone because you may view asking for psychological help as a weakness. It is, actually, a sign of greater strength to say, "This thing is bigger than I can manage alone. I should get some help."

Jenny managed coping with surgery for melanoma because she was good at turning on her "crisis mode" to get her through, but the worries got out of hand when the acute crisis was over:

Jenny, a thirty-seven-year-old investment banker, came to see me after removal of a malignant melanoma from her right calf. Jenny was used to making deals with clients around the world in the middle of the night. She prided herself on thriving on the pressure of stress and competition. Jenny found that the operation was a piece of cake to get through, and she kept her fears about having the melanoma controlled very well. But following her surgery, she was shocked to discover that her usually alert mind couldn't stay focused on her work. During a phone call or at a meeting, thoughts would turn over and over in her mind: "Did they get it all? Am I *really* okay? What are the chances it will come back? Who do I tell that I had a melanoma removed from my leg? Do I tell my boss? I look fine—who's going to believe that I had a malignant tumor removed and that it could come back? Do I need to tell my first serious boyfriend, just as we seem to be possibly making it together?"

Although the pathologist's report gave her a clean bill of health, Jenny did not feel reassured that all the cancer had been removed. The unwanted, repetitive thoughts began to keep her awake much of the night, and she began to feel panicky at times, as if she would have to scream or leave a meeting without explanation. When Jenny and I started to talk, we quickly recognized that she needed to keep busy because this had always been her way of coping with difficulties. However, to do that, she had to get some sleep at night. She began to take an antianxiety medication at bedtime to help her sleep. She awakened more rested in the morning and could concentrate on her work more easily. With rest, her anxious feelings during the day diminished.

I suggested that Jenny get a tape from which she could learn relaxation techniques, so that at night and whenever she felt the panic coming on, she could help herself to relax, stay calm, and put the nagging thoughts out of her mind. We also worked together on her concerns about the prognosis of her melanoma. She talked with her doctor and found out that the melanoma had not extended into the skin or muscle, meaning that it had a high likelihood of not coming back. She debated at length the "who to tell" question and found that, given her personality, she would not do well to keep it a secret. She told her boyfriend, friends, and people at work in a matter-of-fact manner. She was surprised when they responded in the same way, without undue concern. Her anxiety lessened, she began to sleep without medication, and she soon returned to her budding relationship and her vigorous work schedule.

Because there is no "one-size-fits-all" approach to coping with cancer, there is also no one type of counseling that works for everybody. The type of counseling that works best for *you* will depend on several factors. For example, if you are a private person and like to talk only in confidence, individual counseling will probably suit you best. If you opt for individual psychotherapy, approaches abound today, varying from crisis-oriented and supportive to psychodynamic. If you like talking with others in the same situation about shared problems, then a group setting will probably be your cup of tea.

CHOOSING A COUNSELOR AND A TYPE OF THERAPY

The professional you go to for individual or group therapy may be trained primarily in social work, nursing, psychology, psychiatry, or pastoral counseling. The person you select must be skilled in doing psychotherapy and should recognize the need to be flexible, using the approach best suited to the stage of your illness or your particular problem. In a medical crisis, the focus is on the here and now. Supportive therapy is best when illness requires understanding, empathy, and just "being there" from the counselor. People who have returned to health after cancer treatment, however, are often more interested in working on their problems through psychodynamic approaches, which focus on understanding the role of personality and past experiences in emotional reactions and behavior.

I recommend that you find a therapist or counselor who has had experience in treating people with cancer. The psychological problems you face have a sense of urgency not associated with other conditions. The urgency comes from the fact that you are facing a threat to your life. Ideally, your counselor should have worked with oncology teams in the hospital or office and should know about cancer prognoses, treatments, and side effects. For example, fatigue can be caused by cancer or its treatment. It can also be caused by depression. Your therapist has to be able to recognize the difference, perhaps with the help of consultation with the medical team.

Choose a therapist with whom you feel you can talk comfortably. The chemistry or rapport you feel with a particular therapist may be more important than the specific mode of therapy. The feeling of connectedness is key.

Beware of the therapist who tells you that you caused your cancer or that psychotherapy alone will cure it, encouraging you to stop your medical treatment. Therapy plays a remarkably strong role in coping and in ensuring that you get the best treatment, but proof of its direct effect on tumor growth is still missing, and it is never a substitute for medical treatment.

WHAT'S GOOD ABOUT ONE-ON-ONE COUNSELING?

"The therapist is like a sounding board."

"I have someone with whom I can express my worst fears without burdening my family with them."

"I can talk about regrets I have about how I've lived my life, without upsetting the persons I love most."

"My therapist reassures me that I'm not crazy— that the thoughts I have are normal."

"I no longer feel so isolated now, so that I can share how I feel with someone else."

SOME PERSONAL STORIES

Some people find that a cancer diagnosis dredges up suppressed feelings about long-kept secrets from the past. This is especially true of acts associated with guilt, which would hurt others if revealed. The burden of past guilt or shame that surfaces when life is threatened is often lessened by psychotherapy, which puts it into perspective.

After surgery for a kidney tumor, Nancy came to me for help. A devout Roman Catholic, she was devoted to her husband and two children. "I've become so upset and guilty that I'm not able to sleep," she began. "My husband can't understand why I'm not content and happy since I'm doing okay as far as the cancer is concerned. People keep saying, 'You didn't deserve a thing like this.' Down deep I keep feeling that I *did* deserve this cancer. I have lived for years with the guilt that, ten years ago, I became involved with my boss. I broke it off, and my husband never knew. I've never told anyone about it before. I had put it away in a part of my brain so I could live with it, but now I keep feeling maybe this is God's way of punishing me, and the cancer will come back again. I can't stop this thought—it keeps going over and over in my mind."

Nancy and I discussed this fear and her guilt over several sessions. She did believe that her God was loving and forgiving and that her fear of punishment seemed irrational at times. But it still disturbed her. With Nancy's permission, I consulted the Catholic chaplain who belongs to Memorial's multifaith chaplaincy service. He agreed to see her. Through sharing this painful secret with him as a representative of her faith, Nancy was able to resolve her guilt and regain peace in her life. He both understood her pain and could offer forgiveness in the way that was important for Nancy. Our combined psychological and spiritual approach was effective in letting Nancy move on with her life and family.

The diagnosis of cancer, as in Nancy's case, is often a catalyst for resolving old conflicts, both those within ourselves and those that involve others. The existential crisis of cancer evokes the essential question: What if I die? Each person has his or her own way of completing that question: What if I die and never make up with my brother? What if I don't have the chance to apologize to my parents? What can I do *now* to resolve the problems with my daughter? I can't leave with things as they are. These issues suddenly become acute, whereas formerly they could wait with the ready assumption, "One day I'll take care of that."

The case of Gail, an older woman who had completed her treatment for stomach cancer, is a touching example of how counseling can help:

Gail was a very insightful woman with a strong character. She asked to see me because she had always been the linchpin in the family. Her husband was less mature than she and had a bad temper, which had always hampered his relationship with her and the children. Gail's ability to help her husband and the children in facing her death was impaired by his refusal to acknowledge that she was gravely ill. He insisted on treating her as if nothing were wrong, refusing to talk about it. In an emotional session with the couple, her husband finally expressed his fears, saying he could not imagine life without her. Over several weeks, they became closer than they had been in many years.

With this accomplished, Gail could deal with her deeper concern, that of helping her adult children face her likely fatal outcome. "I want to be able to talk with them honestly, try to help them deal with my death, and be a model for them in how to face it."

Sometimes, the existential crisis of cancer is a catalyst for making long-delayed painful decisions:

Joan was a young woman of thirty-five who had divorced an abusive husband when her son was two. A teacher, she managed as a single mother and fully expected to raise her son alone. When her son was six, she developed lung cancer. The tumor was caught early, and her prognosis was good. Nevertheless, she realized that she had to make an alternative plan for her son in case of her death. Several sessions of counseling helped her to get the legal assistance she needed and to approach her brother, who had children of the same

age and whom she trusted to love her son. She also wrote a
will, with her lawyer's help, that ensured her wishes would
be carried out. Having taken care of this important obligation, she could go on with her daily activities with the sense
that her son's future was secure. Although Joan's cancer has
not recurred and her prognosis is excellent, she feels that her
decision to come to terms with the issue of custody for her
son has brought her peace of mind and allayed her anxiety
about the cancer's coming back.

At times, it seems receiving a cancer diagnosis is just part of the
"double troubles" that some people experience. Life's problems
don't seem to get doled out in tolerable and equally divided doses;
often it seems cancer is only part of a double dose of stress. For
example, I've seen cancer develop in an older husband who was taking care of his chronically ill wife, at a time when their income had
plummeted with retirement. Supportive counseling in their home
was extremely helpful to them, along with a social worker's assistance in getting a visiting nurse and a home health aide for them. I
always marvel at how remarkably well people shoulder the heavy
burdens added to their lives by cancer. I often point this out since
people usually think how poorly, not how well, they are managing.
    Another great relief brought about by counseling is the oppor-
tunity to express your true feelings, even the "unacceptable" ones.

Dorothy, a woman in her sixties, came to see me during her
chemotherapy for breast cancer, following a mastectomy.
Her single daughter had taken leave from a highly responsible job in the West to come stay with her. Dorothy came to
my office feeling depressed and guilty because she was so
irritable with her daughter. As she talked, she realized that
she felt so bad because her daughter had sacrificed her work
to come and help her. But in point of fact, she much pre-
ferred to be alone; her daughter made her feel she was more
ill and helpless than was indeed the case. Moreover, the two
of them had a long history of "pushing each other's buttons."
I met with the daughter, who sensed the problem but feared,

because her mother was so ill, that this might be her only chance to make things up to her and somehow to resolve her own guilt about prior problems. A few sessions with the two of them together clarified that the mother was tolerating the chemotherapy well and wanted and needed to be more independent. The daughter also came to understand that her overcompensation for guilt was not necessary.

Amid some tears and laughter, they hugged and agreed that their relationship was truly their own and, indeed, that they did best with each other when each "had her own space." The daughter went back to her home on the West Coast, and return visits are a pleasure for both of them.

PROBLEM SOLVING

This is a simple but highly effective way of helping people deal with cancer. It asks you to look at the problem at hand and to change the way you look at it so that it becomes more tolerable. You "reframe" the problem in your mind. For example, if you have a new pain after an operation for cancer, you might immediately assume it is a sign that the cancer has returned or is probably progressing. You don't stop to think of all the other highly likely reasons it could be there. By helping you to focus objectively on the pain and recognize that, indeed, it is likely nothing, you have changed the way you view it and reduced your distress.

Another example of how you can use this problem-solving approach (cognitive reframing) arises when you're overwhelmed by something and feel you have no control over it. Reframing says, "Break up the problem into little pieces, and tackle one piece at a time." This gets rid of the terrible feeling, "Oh my God, how will I ever get through this!" For instance, you're supposed to start three months of weekly chemotherapy treatments, and this seems like an impossible undertaking for you. But if you look at the whole as a series of tasks, it's easier. First, think of learning the facts about your particular treatment. Afterward, you can meet the chemotherapy nurse and become familiar with the setting of the treatment (getting comfortable in the chair and with other routine aspects). Then you can focus on getting through the initial chemotherapy cycle, and nothing more. Cope with one day at a time. By dealing intellectually with each part of the whole experience, instead of worrying about the entire three months at one time, you can harness your emotional and psychological energies. In this type of problem solving, you use cognitive powers to think and act in ways that carry you through what you want to accomplish. Learning to see difficulties as problems to solve gives you a set of skills that you can apply to other situations in your life.

SEXUAL COUNSELING

Many survivors of cancer have sexual problems that come from physical changes related to surgery, chemotherapy, or radiation, as well as from the emotional baggage that comes with cancer. Considerable research has explored the nature of these difficulties so that professionals know more about them and can do more to help with them today.

If you have had a sexual problem after cancer treatments, you know how hard it is to bring up the topic with the doctor. And you also know that the doctor rarely asks if you have any sexual concerns. The result is that you leave the office without discussing the problem and without getting advice about it. You must forget your embarrassment and describe your sexual concerns. If you need more advice, ask for a referral to a sexual or couples counselor who can deal with both the physical and emotional issues; the two are intertwined and must be addressed together. Sarah Auchincloss, a psychiatrist in my group who is trained in both psycho-oncology and sexual counseling, offers a helpful summary of the problems faced by cancer survivors and encountered in one or more of the three physiological phases of sexual response: desire, excitement, and orgasm.

Desire, including sexual thoughts, fantasies, and interest in sex, is usually low during the period of active treatment for cancer. Less sexual desire in you and your partner comes from being preoccupied with the frightening reality of cancer, its treatment, and its threat to life itself. Other causes of lower desire are premature menopause in women, low-to-absent testosterone in men, and fatigue in both men and women.

In the excitement phase, men may have trouble getting or sustaining an erection. These problems are common after pelvic surgery or radiation in men for bladder, prostate, and colorectal cancer. A urologist who specializes in penile prostheses can explain the available types and the implantation procedure. Viagra has not proved helpful in these situations. (See Chapter 8 for information on genitourinary cancer and sexual therapy.)

For women, dryness and soreness in the vagina, which may lead to painful intercourse, often is treated effectively with local or oral estrogens (when not contraindicated) and vaginal lubricants. Surgery and radiation to the pelvis and chemotherapy cause damage to the ovaries, resulting in these symptoms. Vaginal dilators may help prevent narrowing of the vagina from scarring or fibrosis from the radiation or surgery. If you are in a relationship, couples therapy can help to guide you gradually to more pleasurable sexual functioning by addressing the physical and psychological issues and encouraging you and your partner to work together on the issues.

The case of Margaret, a forty-five-year-old teacher, illustrates the benefits of sexual counseling after cancer treatment:

Margaret was leading a full life, balancing her time between career, home, and family, when a routine Pap smear revealed she had cervical cancer. She was treated with radiation therapy, which offered a high likelihood of cure. During her treatment, she and her husband were so worried about her illness that they didn't think about sex. However, after treatment, Margaret discovered that her sexual feelings were returning. The first few times she and her husband attempted intercourse, Margaret found it painful. Out of anxiety, she began to avoid lovemaking, which her husband interpreted as rejection. He then stopped approaching her, which she believed meant that he was repulsed by her because of her illness.

Eventually, the couple realized that the sexual issue was responsible for a growing distance between them. They consulted a sex counselor, who felt that Margaret's fear of pain during intercourse was the problem. The counselor offered exercises and advice for reducing both her pain and her anxiety. In a couple of months, their sexual life and marriage returned to normal, with a bonus. They had gained a heightened appreciation for each other by successfully confronting a challenge together.

The orgasm phase for both men and women may be inhibited by anxiety, depression, fatigue, and treatment side effects. Pelvic surgery for testicular cancer causes nerve damage resulting in little or no ejaculation, but erectile function is normal. Operations for colon, bladder, and prostate cancer can sometimes cut nerves that control erection, leading to partial or complete impotence. Hormonal treatment for prostate cancer leads to elimination of testosterone and impotence. Referral to a urologist who specializes in penile implants is helpful. Sildenafil (Viagra) is likely of limited value. Psychological factors can also affect sexual response; a sex or couples counselor can identify anxiety or fear of failure as the cause of the problem and advise on ways to show affection and achieve intimacy with oral and manual stimulation.

The American Cancer Society publishes excellent books on sexuality and cancer, one for men and one for women. The author of both is Leslie Schover, a psychologist and researcher on problems of sexual dysfunction in cancer survivors (see Resources at the end of the book).

GROUP PSYCHOTHERAPY

By far the most readily available type of psychological help for people with cancer is support groups. For many years, there was a consensus among those working with cancer patients that it was not desirable for patients to talk with one another. "They'll be comparing their treatments and doctors." "What will happen when one dies? Won't that make it harder?" The evidence from experience is strongly to the contrary. The first support groups were sponsored by the American Cancer Society after World War II, and they were organized for people who had lost a major function, such as speech. By the 1960s, patients themselves began grassroots efforts, forming self-help groups to deal with special problems. As women became more assertive with the advent of the feminist movement, they started support and advocacy groups to increase attention to the psychological aspects of breast cancer.

Today, there is almost a "tyranny of groups": People are criticized if they don't join one. Families worry that "Uncle John is refusing to go to a group; he isn't fighting his cancer." My point is, again, that we're all different. Groups are great for some people but terrible for others. My advice is to go a few times and see how it feels. If it is frightening and makes you feel worse, don't go back. If you are the type of person who takes a while to warm up to new people and situations, you may want to give the group time to see if it feels better.

The best contact for identifying groups in your locality is the American Cancer Society, which is usually aware of the self-help groups, including where they are located and how to contact them. Many are free; others are covered by health insurance including Medicare.

There are different types of groups. Some groups are run by a professional, whereas self-help groups are led by patients themselves. Some groups are open to patients with all types of cancer; others limit participation to people with the same type of cancer, for example, breast or prostate cancer. Some groups are geared toward people at a particular stage of life and, consequently, grappling with specific issues, such as the groups we offer for young adults and for adults over age fifty at Memorial. Some groups are closed and meet for a fixed number of times; others are open so that people can come and go as they choose. Time-limited groups provide helpful support for patients, but the downside is that it's hard to stop when you have found something that makes you feel better; you may feel a void in your life once the group stops meeting. Sharing telephone numbers and having follow-up meetings encourage continued contact. Some groups invite family members. The Wellness Community, Gilda's Clubs, Cancer Care, Y-Me, and Us Too are national organizations that offer groups for patients and survivors (see Resources).

I have worked in a group format with patients with lung cancer over the past two years, and we have had a good chance to explore the positives and negatives of being in such a group. The positives are clear. There is an immediate sense of being in a room where every-body knows what everyone else is going through. Members have said things like this: "We're all coping with exactly the same prob-lems. Outside this group, it's like I'm in another country, I feel so different from healthy people." "I feel I can say what I really feel here. I don't have to censor what I say like I do at home to spare my family."

The stigma of having cancer is reduced by group support. "People look at me as if they don't know what to say," said Ron, a fifty-six-year-old construction foreman with lung cancer. "They seem to be saying, 'You brought it on yourself by smoking, and we all know what a serious disease lung cancer is.'" The sense of being different and ostracized is real, but the comaraderie of the group helps offset it.

Doctors and treatments are big topics in cancer support groups. You can compare notes on available treatments and to compare which treatments are being used by different doctors and centers. You also feel free to criticize the doctors and the "medical system." "Would you believe what my doctor said!" is followed by laughter and the sense of relief that comes from sharing. But the other side is expressed also. Instances of the kindness or tenderness expressed by a doctor or nurse are told with appreciative reflection. Individuals gain the confidence to speak more assertively with their doctors and navigate their way through managed care as a result of hearing how others do it.

Another big topic discussed in the group is complementary and alternative therapies. The group setting permits a comfortable opportunity to share information and talk about ideas that a medical team might dismiss or disparage. Seeking out alternatives like Chinese herbs, food supplements, mind-body techniques, and acupuncture meets the need people have to "do something" for themselves (see Chapter 10).

The group often focuses on how loved ones are faring and how best to handle them. Patients often feel guilty for "upsetting the applecart" of their family's lives. Many also strongly dislike having to ask others for help and have a particularly hard time facing a loss of independence. Most worry a lot about their family's future welfare "in case I don't make it." This topic is often hard to raise with family members because they may misinterpret it as Mom or Dad is giving up, while talking about the issue could bring you peace of mind.

> Barbara developed lung cancer at sixty-five. She had lost her husband a year earlier to a massive heart attack, which destroyed their happily planned retirement together. She told the group of this enormous disappointment and also shared her fear of facing illness alone. Her children were busy with their lives. She felt they cared, but they really didn't have time to accompany her to doctors' visits. How much should Barbara expect of the children? How should she talk with her grandchildren, ages fourteen and ten, about her illness? She didn't want to alarm them, but she also felt they needed to know about her situation. She wanted to prepare them for the fact that she could die. The group made the connections between her problem and their own situations. They supported her asking her children to come to her home after a chemotherapy treatment to bring her things she needed and cook simple foods for her. They agreed that the children and grandchildren should be told and kept abreast of how she was feeling.
>
> To her surprise, the children rallied to help her when she finally got the courage to ask them. Her daughter arranged her schedule so that she could go to the doctors' visits, and sitting together in the waiting room proved to be an opportunity to talk and to draw closer to each other.

Treatment decisions are often shared in groups. In Stages III and IV disease, treatments are frequently varied and involve experimental therapies. Being told that "there is no accepted, surefire treatment" for your cancer is frightening. Also, it is hard to decide whether to accept whatever new chemotherapy or radiation treatment is being offered. However, hearing how others fared while on the same shaky ground can be extremely helpful and reassuring.

Group discussions are often a forum for expressing anger. The anger can be about having cancer, the doctor, the side effects of the treatment, the unpleasant wait at the doctor's office, insensitive behavior of office staff, behavior and attitudes of healthy people, lack of adequate resources to find cures in time to help, and the sense of urgency about life that isn't understood by others. A group is a good place to vent feelings that are sometimes labeled as irrational by others. Within the group, these frustrations are accorded respect and are accepted with empathy.

What are the downsides to being in a group? It's hard to see others who are less ill ("I wish I were as well as he"). It can be even harder to see someone who is sicker than you ("I just look at her and worry that I'll be that sick soon"). For some, this knowledge can be reassuring ("It's better to be aware of all the possibilities and deal with them in someone else"). Of course, it is profoundly sad to lose a friend in the group. Relationships become close, and grieving for a lost member is painful. However, as noted by members of Dr. David Spiegel's support group in Stanford, "talking about death detoxifies it" and makes it less threatening.

These downsides are too hard for some people; for them, the distress exceeds the benefits of the group. If you are one of these individuals, I encourage you to talk privately with someone, and don't feel bad if you find the group too upsetting for you.

Those who benefit from groups look forward to each session and find the advice, as well as the company, comforting and uplifting. The friendships that develop among group members provide a critically important link to others who care and understand. Most cancers develop in later years when support from one's spouse and friends may be diminishing or absent. The group is particularly good for persons who are alone and who feel isolated. Ties in the group substitute in part for missing family members.

Even for those who have plenty of support at home, however, the group offers an environment where you can be yourself, speak openly, and talk with others "who really know what I'm talking about." You may feel, as David was quoted as saying at the beginning of this chapter, that you're "all in the same leaky boat." For many, cancer support groups are like a lifeboat, in which you ride out the rough waves together.

MIND-BODY TECHNIQUES

One of the most commonly felt and difficult aspects of having cancer is the sense that you no longer have control over your life. Exercises and therapies that you learn and practice yourself give you a renewed sense of control. A range of "self-generated" techniques can be used, which we refer to as *mind-body methods.* Once you learn them, you own them and can use them anytime. Among the more popular are meditation, relaxation exercises, guided imagery, and self-hypnosis. Some people are especially attracted to creative approaches aimed at self-expression, such as art therapy, music therapy, and creative writing or journaling about illness.

By using these valuable methods, you can actually control your distressing symptoms like anxiety, pain, and even nausea. This isn't to say that if any of these symptoms becomes severe, you won't need medication to control it. But there is little doubt that mind-body techniques help you keep your emotions in check. When you are calm, discomfort and pain become more tolerable. Consider the mind-body methods as adjuncts to help you go through your illness.

Achieving the relaxation response is the simplest of these techniques; the response is induced in various ways such as simple deep breathing, conscious relaxation of muscles, and yoga. Choose the approach that works best for you. Some relaxation techniques are described below. Many others are available in books or on tape (see Resources). Alternatively, you can learn them from a health professional at your cancer center or in your community.

Progressive Muscle Relaxation

This most common method teaches you to tense and relax different muscles, consciously, until your entire body feels relaxed. The following is done to a count of three, but you may be able to sustain each movement to a count of four or five as you progress.

1. This exercise is best done lying on your back. If that is not a comfortable position for you, you may do it sitting up in bed, as long as your back is

supported. If you are sitting, you may want to cross your legs.

2. Lying comfortably, become aware of your breathing, which should be kept in a regular, steady pattern.

3. Begin with your hands. Tighten and clench your fists as you slowly count to three: 1, 2, 3. Now let all the tension in your hands go.

4. Now tense the muscles in your feet. Clench your toes to the count of three: 1, 2, 3. At the count of three, let all the tension in your feet go.

5. Now move up the body to your legs. Tense your calves and thighs. Hold for a count of three. At three, let your legs go limp.

6. Continue to move up the body to your torso. Pull in your stomach muscles, tighten your chest: 1, 2, 3. (Remember: Don't strain yourself, and don't tense any area that's sore or painful.) Let your chest and abdomen relax. Take a few deep breaths, and let them out long. Let your breathing return to normal before proceeding.

7. Now tense your shoulders. Count: 1, 2, 3. Let your shoulders soften and relax totally.

8. Now move up to your neck. Tense up your neck muscles: 1, 2, 3. Now let all the tension out of your neck. Take a few deep breaths, and let them out. Let your breathing return to its normal rate.

9. Now focus on your face. Close your eyes tightly. Count: 1, 2, 3. Now release all tension from your eyes, and gently open them.

10. Tighten your forehead: 1, 2, 3. Release all tension from your forehead.

11. Crinkle your nose. Count: 1, 2, 3. Relax your nose.

12. Make a big smile, and hold it for three seconds. Then let your mouth relax.

13. Now tighten all the muscles of your face, making a funny face. Hold it for a count of three: 1, 2, 3. Now relax all your facial muscles.

14. Tense up your entire body. Count: 1, 2, 3. Let your entire body relax. Now lie still for a few moments. If you feel tension in any part of your body, try to tighten the muscles in that area gently and then gently release the tension. Relax, as you breathe as peacefully as you can, and remain in this relaxed state for several minutes.

DEEP BREATHING

Many spiritual disciplines use breathing exercises to focus the mind and promote relaxation. The old adage "take a deep breath and count to ten" to help you remain in control in difficult situations has strong scientific roots. This technique is simple, and you can apply it anywhere and anytime. Some people use it to calm down in the dentist's or doctor's waiting room before a scary procedure.

The following is a simple deep-breathing exercise; you can pace yourself when you try it. It starts with a short breath, breathing in for only one count, and builds up to a count of five. If you feel short of breath or don't have the stamina to go all the way to a count of five, stop. Find your own comfort level.

1. Close your eyes. Take a breath in, on the count of one, and breathe out on the count of one.

2. Now take a slightly deeper breath while counting to two. Let the breath out while counting to two.

3. Take the breath in a little longer, counting to three, and let the breath out to the count of three.

4. Now deepen the breath to the count of four, and exhale to the count of four.

5. Breathe in to the count of five, and breathe out to the count of five.

6. Now gradually work back down from five counts to four, then to three, then to two, and then to one.

7. Let your breathing return to its natural rhythm. Sit quietly for a few moments.

Here is a simple way to count out this breathing exercise:

1
Breathe in: 1. Breathe out: 1.

2
Breathe in: 1, 2. Breathe out: 1, 2.

3
Breathe in: 1, 2, 3. Breathe out: 1, 2, 3.

4
Breathe in: 1, 2, 3, 4. Breathe out: 1, 2, 3, 4.

5
Breathe in: 1, 2, 3, 4, 5. Breathe out: 1, 2, 3, 4, 5.

6
Breathe in: 1, 2, 3, 4. Breathe out: 1, 2, 3, 4.

7
Breathe in: 1, 2, 3. Breathe out: 1, 2, 3.

8

Breathe in: 1, 2. Breathe out: 1, 2.

9

Breathe in: 1. Breathe out: 1.

10

Breathe normally, and sit quietly for a short while.

You can vary this breathing exercise by adding an image or a color to the count. For instance, breathe in picturing a soothing aqua blue color, then breathe out. Breathe in and picture a tranquil mountain. Breathe out.

HYPNOSIS

Most of us who work with people who are ill view hypnosis as a technique that lets you reach a deep level of relaxation in which you become less aware of your environment. Only people who want to experience an altered state of consciousness and who respond well to suggestion can actually do so. Some people are reluctant to try hypnosis because they are afraid they will lose control. In fact, this technique is helpful to control anxiety and to relieve mild pain.

In one innovative strategy that works well for children, the therapist or parent guides the child in creating a tale or imagery in which the character triumphs over the child's fears. The child identifies with the heroine or hero and feels self-assertive, proud, and secure. The feared objects, like needle sticks, are brought into the story by the therapist. This technique works because children love to make believe. Dr. William Redd recounted the story of Ricky.

Ricky, a seven-year-old boy with leukemia, had a terrible fear of needles. When it was his turn to go into the treatment room, he would kick, scream, and hide under a chair, holding on with all his strength. To help the boy keep his mind off the needle and stay calm, a therapist made up a story about Batman and Robin.

"One time, Batman and Robin went on a trip and found an invisible magic glove. Anybody who wore it became strong and could withstand any pain. One day

Robin asked Batman if he could borrow the magic glove for a doctor's visit, because Robin didn't like getting shots. Batman lent Robin the glove, and when Robin got a shot, he didn't feel a thing."

The therapist then put the invisible magic glove on Ricky's hand. From then on, Ricky always put on the magic glove before his chemotherapy. To the relief of his parents and nurses, this greatly reduced his terror. In fact, when he saw another child crying one day before his shot, he asked, "Mommy, can I give *him* my magic glove?"

MEDITATION

Most of the time, you probably focus on things outside of yourself: work, family, friends, and errands. Meditation is just the opposite. It demands that you concentrate your attention totally within yourself. To meditate, you must think only of the present moment and of your body, focusing on breathing. You may focus on a special word or phrase, a prayer, or an image that produces a relaxed, calm, and serene feeling.

Meditation can be a spiritual or a wholly secular experience. Some form of meditation is found in virtually every spiritual and religious tradition. However you choose to use it, you may find it helpful. Studies by Dr. Jon Kabat-Zinn, psychologist at the University of Massachusetts at Worcester, and others have shown that meditation reduces both physical pain and distress. If you practice it frequently, you may find that you have a new sense of calmness that you didn't have before.

The mindfulness meditation of Tibetan Buddhists is used by Dr. David Payne, a psychologist in my group at Memorial, who works with behavioral and spiritual approaches. In his Journey to the Moment group, Payne teaches this method, giving instructions to use awareness of breathing as a way to focus your thoughts on your body and on the present moment, brushing away thoughts of the past and future.

A method is outlined for you here. It is best to start doing meditation for five to ten minutes and gradually build up to a longer period of time (thirty minutes or more). Select a special place that is quiet, where you will not be disturbed. Once you have established a practice routine, try to meditate for at least twenty minutes. Some people like to meditate at night to help themselves go to sleep. Others start the day with it.

Here are two simple methods of meditating that you may wish to try:

MEDITATION ON THE BREATH

1. Choose a quiet place where you are unlikely to be distracted by noises.

2. Posture: You can meditate in any steady yet comfortable posture, including lying down, sitting in a chair, sitting up in bed, or sitting cross-legged on the floor.

   If you are lying down, either in bed, on the floor, or on a mat, you may wish to place a pillow under your head for comfort.

   If you are sitting up in bed, place a pillow or cushion behind your back.

   If you are sitting in a chair, place your feet on the floor. If your feet do not reach the floor, place them on a pillow or cushion.

   If you are sitting on the floor, sit on a cushion, pillow, or rolled-up blanket, so that your "sit-bones" are higher than your knees. If your knees are uncomfortable, place a cushion or blanket beneath them.

3. Close your eyes.

4. Take a deep breath, and let it out slowly. Repeat this two more times, inhaling deeply and exhaling slowly. Then let your breathing return to its normal pattern.

5. Focus your attention on your breath. Be aware of your breath going in and going out. As thoughts come up in your mind, put them aside, thinking of them as clouds moving across the sky. Return to awareness of your breathing.

6. Sit quietly like this for a short while.

7. When you are ready to end your meditation, take a deep inhalation and let out a long exhalation. (You may wish to repeat this once or twice more.) Then let your breathing return to normal, and when you are ready, open your eyes. It helps to set a timer for the end of the session since it is hard to guess the time when you are meditating; time passes much faster than you think.

SPECIAL WORD MEDITATION

Another common form of meditation is to focus your attention on a word, phrase, or prayer. In yoga, this type of meditation is called *mantra meditation*.

1. Choose your "special word." This can be any word that has a meaning for you, such as love, peace, or harmony. If you like, you can choose a word or phrase from your religious tradition or cultural heritage, for example, a phrase from the Lord's Prayer or the word *shalom* (Hebrew for "peace"). Or you can pick a simple word, such as *one*.

2. Close your eyes. Take a deep breath and let it out long. Repeat this two more times, taking in a deep inhalation, followed by a long exhalation.

3. Begin to repeat your special word silently to yourself at your natural rate of speaking.

4. If you have chosen a short word or phrase, you may wish to coordinate it with your breathing—for example, breathing in as you say the word to yourself, and then breathing out as you say the word again. Or you may visualize a symbol to go with the word, such as a sunrise, calm lake, or clear moon.

5. Continue to repeat the word, phrase, or prayer to yourself throughout the time you have allotted for your meditation.

6. When thoughts arise that distract you, simply bring your mental awareness back to your special word or phrase and continue to repeat it.

7. When it is time to end your meditation, take a deep breath and let it out, repeating this one or two times. When you are ready, open your eyes.

GUIDED IMAGERY

Imagery simply means finding an image or picture in your mind that you associate with a feeling of well-being and peace. A mountain stream with rushing waters and biking on a beach at sunset are two examples. Audiotapes are available offering a vast range of possible images. This is a technique you can use to distract your thoughts from a particular unpleasant or frightening situation or feeling. The technique may be used with relaxation methods as well as hypnosis.

Some patients with cancer choose to use the image of the cells of their immune system killing off the cancer cells. Others say, "It frightens me to death to picture something like that." Use any approach that makes you feel comfortable. We don't have any evidence that the immune system works better when you visualize the cells, but if the imagery promotes a sense of calmness that your body is working for you, that in itself is worthwhile. Create your own images that make you feel calm and relaxed.

Close your eyes. Begin your imagery with a relaxation exercise you like. Once you feel relaxed, imagine that you are in a beautiful, calm setting. For example, picture yourself floating on a raft in the middle of a cool lake, if that appeals to you. The water beneath you is still, with barely a ripple. The sky is a clear, pale blue. White clouds slowly drift across it. Birds fly by overhead, singing. Your body rocks gently and peacefully on the water. Continue to breathe at your natural rate and to picture this scene.

Envision any natural setting that appeals to you, such as a beautiful forest, a field of fragrant flowers, a beach, or a mountain. You will likely picture yourself in a favorite place where you have spent enjoyable times. Imagine the scene with all your senses. Answer these questions:

> What does it look like?

> What sounds do I hear?

> How does my body feel? Is there a warm sun overhead, or a cool refreshing breeze, for instance?

> Is there a particular fragrance or aroma in the air?

> Do I associate a particular taste with this place?

While imagining this place, notice your calmness and improved emotional state When you are ready to end your guided imagery exercise, take a deep breath and let it out long. Open your eyes.

Imagery has been called the language of the feeling brain. It sharpens all your senses. Relaxation with guided imagery and meditation helps you stay calm during frightening procedures, like an MRI or a bone marrow aspiration. Although these techniques derive from Eastern spiritual traditions, some of the effects are similar to those obtained from counseling and psychotherapy: focusing the mind, increasing self-awareness, and enhancing a sense of mastery.

SPIRITUALITY AND PASTORAL COUNSELING

Spirituality takes many forms. For some people, spirituality is their personal search for meaning, however that quest evolves. For others, spirituality represents a philosophy of life that gives transcendent meaning to life and death. But in all of its forms, spirituality enables people to develop a perspective in which they feel better able to cope with unavoidable suffering and to come to terms with personal tragedy and loss. Some people adopt a secular philosophy of life, which has worked for them in the past and helped them through life crises. Personal beliefs are acquired and finely honed over a lifetime. Having something to "hold on to," whatever belief system it is, seems to sustain people during a crisis of serious illness. I see my work as helping people to identify the belief or philosophy of life that has served them well in the past and to apply this inner reservoir of support to their present crisis. My colleagues and I never try to change anyone's personal beliefs.

Gallup polls in the United States show that 96 percent of people believe in God, but less than half attend religious services. Many people who grew up in a religious tradition left it in their adult life. But illness is an existential crisis that often prompts us to reexplore spiritual roots, as we seek to find meaning in the face of a threat to life and possible death. When we find we have no answers, we go looking for them, often in old, familiar forms. More than 70 percent of patients surveyed at Memorial Sloan-Kettering Cancer Center indicated that they used prayer in coping with their illness. Like meditation, prayer releases emotions and leads to a calmer state of mind. For many people, prayer, meditation, and reading from sacred and philosophical sources are deeply comforting.

Counseling from a member of the clergy of your faith is a helpful resource. Pastoral counseling may help you to sort out vexing questions, like "If God is good and loves me, how can He allow this to happen to me?" or "Am I being punished now for my past sins?" or "What can I hope for?" At the center of all pastoral counseling is the effort to help you marshal hope in facing suffering and an uncertain future. Daniel Callahan, an ethicist at the Hastings Center, wrote:

> Hope accepts painful facts, but seeks to place them in a broader perspective that includes other, more acceptable aspects of those facts.

Hope, to be authentic, must be based on reality, taking into account the obvious meaning of a tragic or life-threatening event, but then it seeks other perspectives that people welcome, for example, finding meaning in "transcendent hope."

Often in the face of illness, the spiritual side of people reaches out beyond the differences among religious groups. Father Tom McDonnell, a Catholic priest and psychologist at Memorial, chose to work at night because, he said, "Things are always worse and more frightening for patients when it's dark." He tells of a night when a Hasidic Jewish mother was sitting outside the Surgical Recovery Unit awaiting news of the outcome of her son's surgery. The mother became very concerned when the door opened and she saw that her son's yarmulke (skullcap) was not on his head. In her worry and fear, it was important that this symbol of her religion be observed. Father Tom asked the mother for the yarmulke and reverently placed it on her son's head as he lay sleeping. Then the Catholic priest and the Hasidic mother sat together and prayed. The power of faith in both traditions joined in a single act of healing prayer for a mother's son.

CREATIVE THERAPIES

Some people have a hard time expressing their fears orally and gain the most solace from nontalking therapies. Some examples of these expressive methods are described in this section.

JOURNALING

Keeping a diary or journal can bring clarity and perspective to your experiences, while providing a vehicle for expressing your feelings about your illness. In itself, this can be cathartic. Dr. James W. Pennebaker, a psychologist at the University of Texas, has written about the therapeutic value of expressing emotions on paper. According to Pennebaker, in his book *Opening Up: The Healing Power of Expressing Emotions*, the mere act of talking or writing about upsetting experiences "can change the ways we think and feel about traumatic events, and about ourselves."

In research studies, Pennebaker and his colleagues found that students who wrote "their deepest thoughts and feelings" about traumas had a more positive outlook, improved mood (less depression), and even better physical health than those who wrote about superficial events. (For example, the students who wrote about their traumas made fewer visits to the student health center.) Moreover, in a study with psychologist Janice Kiecolt-Glaser and immunologist Ronald Glaser of Ohio State University, Pennebaker found that the immune function of people who wrote about deep feelings related to an earlier traumatic experience was better than that of people who wrote about superficial topics.

You may find writing about your experiences with illness a helpful way to identify feelings, record them, and then look back at them later, as did Cornelius Ryan and Kathlyn Conway (described in Chapters 4 and 11, respectively).

ART PSYCHOTHERAPY

At Memorial, Paola Luzzatto, a psychologist and an art therapist, has been exploring the use of art forms to help patients with cancer express their anger, vulnerability, loss, fears, and depression. She has found that some people gain comfort from working in groups and sharing the meaning of the images they have created. Others prefer private sessions with her. Luzzatto believes that the most deeply buried feelings of pain and fear are released in these sessions in ways that would never have been possible using words. Art psychotherapy allows you to "draw the pain," that is, illustrate your pain through an image or symbol, as well as explore its meaning for you. In expressing your pain through art, you may also reduce its intensity.

Art psychotherapy is not just for those who have artistic talent. This medium invites all who feel isolated or have difficulty communicating in words. It has special value for those who have had surgery that impairs speech and, especially, for those who have lost their voice after the surgical removal of the voice box. It lends itself to all ages and is a particularly successful approach for children with cancer. Finally, art therapy allows you an opportunity to pursue a creative activity when illness precludes more physically demanding ones.

Art psychotherapy also provides a vehicle for "containing," or putting into perspective, some of the overwhelming feelings evoked by cancer. Having a safe way to express feelings that may be too difficult to talk about can be profoundly freeing and soothing. One patient said, "I was relieved of my pent-up anger, and I became more calm."

The freedom of letting yourself go and seeing where your creativity leads you can also boost your self-esteem and your sense of personal control over your circumstances. Drawing or painting can be liberating and exhilarating, especially when you are struggling with new limitations and loss. Without consciously intending to create anything specific, you can find unexpected meanings in your artwork. The chaos, disorder, meaninglessness, and "out-of-control" feeling you have can give way to a sense of order, meaning, and autonomy.

MEDICATIONS TO CONTROL DISTRESS

We all take pride in trying to be strong as we face an illness. But sometimes the problems are so great that you just can't "tough it out," no matter how hard you try. At these rough times, you may need to take a medication to reduce your distress.

Today, many drugs are available to help in managing distress. Table 3 lists the commonly used ones. They are safe when taken under the doctor's supervision. They can help you deal with insomnia, depression, anxiety, and some physical symptoms like fatigue and pain. However, people have so many fears about taking medicines for these problems that they sometimes suffer rather than take a medication that would give them relief. These negative attitudes are barriers to reducing distress. They are part of the stigma attached to everything—and anything—psychological. We see the same attitudes and fears in people considering taking medicines for serious pain. Patients often express these concerns by saying things like this:

"I might be a zombie if I take it. I might get addicted."

"I have cancer, and you can't change that with a pill."

"I have to be strong and face this thing on my own. I don't want a tranquilizer."

"I'd be ashamed if people knew I had to take drugs for my nerves. They might think I'm crazy."

"I'm afraid the medicine you want to give me for my nerves might fight with my cancer medicines."

These statements express legitimate concerns, but they also show some of the stigma and fears people associate with anything they feel might alter their thinking. These fears are unwarranted today in the setting of good total care, and they arise largely out of lack of knowledge regarding the actual medicines we use and their side effects, if any. For example, people's fears of becoming addicted, either to pain medication or psychopharmacologic drugs, are out of proportion to the actual risk of this happening. People who have never had a problem with drugs really don't have to worry about getting addicted. They don't have the type of personality that makes them vulnerable to addiction. Besides, medication is closely monitored by the prescribing physician, and it is stopped when it is no longer needed.

Following are descriptions of several situations in which taking a medication can make an important difference.

POOR SLEEP

Problems and worries always seem worse at night in the darkness. Unable to go to sleep, you may lie awake for hours with frightening thoughts racing out of control. You may fall asleep easily but awaken at 4:00 A.M., and *then* the demons come out. Either way, when the morning comes, you are tired and not eager to get up and face a day of work or treatment, or both. After a week or two of sleep loss every night, the fatigue begins to drag you down. Worries and fears automatically seem worse.

If you are receiving cancer treatment and you can't sleep, it might be because of a medication you are taking. For example, corticosteroids (prednisone, dexamethasone [Decadron]) can make you feel tense, restless, and anxious and make your thoughts race. The same can be said of some drugs used to reduce nausea, such as metoclopramide (Reglan) or prochlorperazine (Compazine). These symptoms are relieved by the beta blocker propranolol (Inderal) or by several antianxiety drugs: clonazepam (Klonopin), lorazepam (Ativan), buspirone (Buspar), alprazolam (Xanax), and nefazodone (Serzone). For anxiety from steroids, drugs like olanzapine (Zyprexa) and risperidone (Risperdal) are useful.

If you are having insomnia that interferes with your ability to function, ask your doctor about a sleep medicine. A number of safe drugs are available: Benadryl, an antihistamine, is safe and helpful. Zolpidem (Ambien) is a safe sedative. Several drugs in the benzodiazepine family are useful: temazepam (Restoril), lorazepam (Ativan), and clonazepam (Klonopin). Chloral hydrate is an old and safe medicine for sleep, which is now available only in liquid form.

If you are depressed and also have trouble sleeping, several antidepressants, given at bedtime, are effective: amitriptyline (Elavil), trazodone (Desyrel), and mirtazapine (Remeron). These medicines provide double benefits, reducing both insomnia at night and depression during the day.

ANXIETY

This is the most common form of distress among people with cancer. It can disrupt your life at work and at home and your ability to cope with your illness. If the anxiety is severe, you need a medication along with counseling. The added help from the medication will enable you to feel more like your "old" self and to get your emotions back on track. You will find you are better able to cope with the crises of the disease on your own. Once you get over these rough spots, the medication can be stopped, safely.

Marie, a forty-five-year-old lawyer, had a routine X ray that revealed a suspicious shadow in her lung. She had had anxiety all her life, with a phobia of being in small, enclosed spaces. Moreover, she had had severe panic attacks that came on without warning since she was a teenager. She dreaded the attacks because they made her breathing difficult and her heart race, and she felt terrified during attacks. Marie had not had any attacks in several years. However, when her doctor recommended that she have a diagnostic MRI scan, she became anxious both about the possibility of cancer and about having a panic attack if she had to be placed in a small metal cylinder and lie still. The next day she did indeed have a panic attack in anticipation of the test. She began to feel there was no way that she could go through with the MRI. She told me that she felt "paralyzed" by these fears. I recommended that she take clonazepam (Klonopin), an antianxiety drug, in the morning and at night. After two days, she felt calmer. As we prepared for the MRI, I reassured Marie that music would be piped in and that she should take a pill a half-hour before the procedure. She got through the test without a panic attack.

Anxiety is also apt to occur before tests that are done every three to six months to see if there is evidence that a tumor that has been successfully treated is regrowing. Libby was one such person:

At fifty-eight and a single mother of two college-age children, Libby was back working in retail sales, having finished treatment with chemotherapy following lumpectomy and radiation for breast cancer. She felt good, had her energy back, and believed that she had "put the cancer behind me."

However, her three-months' checkup abruptly brought the cancer back to center stage in her mind. As the time approached for repeating scans and markers (blood tests that show the presence of a tumor), she became panicked. "What if it comes back? What will I do?" She was referred to me by her oncologist, who thought her fears were far out of proportion to the likelihood of recurrence. We talked together about the stresses of the tests and her fears of not being able to keep her children in college if she became ill again. Libby readily agreed to start taking a mild antianxiety medication, buspirone (Buspar), twice a day. It reduced her panicky feelings and didn't interfere with her work. She got through the tests and was able to stay calm while she awaited the results. Over several months, she learned to control the fears better herself. We stopped the medication and began to talk about her problems over the past ten years that centered on raising her two children alone.

Panic attacks are never fun, but they are especially frightening when you are ill. The sense of being unable to breathe, having a choking sensation, or having your heart beat fast makes you think something might be wrong and that it must be caused by the cancer. Several medicines control panic attacks: clonazepam (Klonopin), fluoxetine (Prozac), paroxetine (Paxil), sertraline (Zoloft), and imipramine (Tofranil).

Anxiety, like insomnia, can be a side effect of your cancer medication, especially of steroids and antinausea drugs. To counter the anxiety caused by these medicines, we prescribe the same drugs listed previously in discussing insomnia.

DEPRESSION

We say "I'm depressed" to cover everything from distress due to bad driving weather to feeling seriously down. But true depression—clinical, full-blown depression—is a serious disorder. Symptoms are encompassing: trouble sleeping, loss of appetite, lack of energy, no libido, no motivation, and no enjoyment of things that ordinarily bring you pleasure. You feel helpless, worthless, and that life isn't worth living. Thoughts of not wanting to live and of suicide are the most serious symptoms The physical symptoms of fatigue can be caused by cancer also, so at times it is hard, in a person who has cancer, to tease out what is caused by cancer and what represents depression. I often say, "It seems to me if we got rid of the part of the fatigue that may be coming from depression, then the part coming from cancer will be more tolerable."

You might say that if you have cancer, you have every reason to be depressed. That's true, but we have learned that changes in the chemistry of the brain also contribute to depression. The antidepressant medicines we have nowadays work on serotonin, which is a naturally occurring brain chemical that affects mood. The most widely used antidepressants today, the selective serotonin reuptake inhibitors (SSRIs), act on the brain to raise the level of serotonin. Several SSRIs are widely used because they improve mood and have few side effects: fluoxetine (Prozac), sertraline (Zoloft), paroxetine (Paxil), and citalopram (Celexa).

Other antidepressants, which are not SSRIs but are also effective, are bupropion (Wellbutrin), nefazodone (Serzone), mirtazapine (Remeron), and venlafaxine (Effexor). If you get any side effects from taking one of these drugs (such as dry mouth, queasy stomach, anxiety, or headache), they are likely to be mild and transient, improving over a few days. However, your sensitivity to the drug and its wide range of possible side effects make it important that you work closely with the doctor who prescribed it for you. You may need to adjust the dose or perhaps change to another drug. A word about stopping a medication: It is best to check with your doctor before you stop taking any medication, since some drugs need to be tapered off rather than stopped abruptly.

Depression is sometimes a side effect of cancer medications, especially interferon, interleukin-2 (IL-2), and steroid drugs such as dexamethasone (Decadron) and prednisone. Both interferon and interleukin-2 typically cause flulike symptoms, including depressed mood, due to their action on the brain. The antidepressant drugs just mentioned are good at countering depression that is related to treatment.

If you have had a depression in the past, you are vulnerable to becoming depressed in the course of being treated for cancer. A colleague recently asked me to see her mother, who had been operated on successfully for cancer of the uterus:

> She described her mother as a worrier and a pessimist who tended to look on the dark side of life. She had had a post-partum depression after the birth of her daughter, now thirty. It was not treated at the time, but she had stayed in bed, tearful and sad, while her husband and mother had cared for the new baby for several months. Slowly, she had resumed her normal activities.
>
> Recently, over the three weeks since her operation, she had become morose, withdrawn, and irritable. She could not come to meals with the family, but stayed alone in her room. She was miserable at her daughter's home, but unable to manage at her own apartment. When she came to see me, she looked sad; her face was drawn, and she told me she just couldn't go on. She had no energy and preferred to lie in bed though she couldn't sleep. "Black" thoughts consumed her, and she felt she would be glad if "a Mack truck hap-pened to run over me." She enjoyed nothing, not even her grandchildren, who had been her pride and joy.
>
> We spoke about her depression after her delivery and she recalled it vividly. She recognized the similarity of symp-toms. We agreed that a medication was needed, and I pre-scribed the antidepressant paroxetine (Paxil) for her to take at night. I encouraged her to try to walk some each day and play some with the children. I spoke with her daughter about quietly trying to interest her in watercolor painting, which had been her favorite avocation in the past.
>
> Over two weeks, she improved and became more active and able to interact with her family. By six weeks, she was able to move back to her apartment.

Tricyclic antidepressants (see Table 3 for the list of names) were first used for depression, but they are helpful also in pain control, particularly for *neuropathic* pain, which is caused by direct irritation of a nerve. This type of pain can be quite severe in some cases.

Numbness, tingling, and pain in the fingers and toes are the result of damage to nerve endings caused by some chemotherapy drugs. In these cases, tricyclic drugs work well, reducing discomfort and pain. Amitriptyline (Elavil), desipramine (Norpramin), imipramine (Tofranil), and nortriptyline (Pamelor) are used in conjunction with stronger pain medications, often permitting a lower dose of narcotic medicines.

> Ingrid was a feisty woman who told me chemotherapy wasn't going to get her down. She was tough and could handle whatever the side effects would be. If this was the cost for escaping scot-free from Hodgkin's disease, so be it. All went well until she developed tingling and numbness in her fingers, toes, and feet. She could stand the fingers, but the sensations in her feet made her unsure of walking. She said, "I'm not sure where my feet are moving. They feel numb, as if needles and pins were sticking into the bottoms." Her doctor recognized her symptom: a peripheral neuropathy (nerve damage) caused by the chemotherapy drug vincristine. We placed Ingrid on amitriptyline (Elavil) at bedtime, which reduced the pain and discomfort and eased her depression. At three months, after completing the chemotherapy, Ingrid had almost normal feeling again in her fingers and feet, and her mood was normal.

Fatigue is extremely common in cancer, and more attention is finally being given to it. It can come from chemotherapy and radiation side effects, which lower red blood cells and cause anemia, or it can be caused by depression. It is important that you tell your doctor if you feel fatigued so that he or she can determine the true cause. If your fatigue is caused by depression, several drugs are very helpful: methylphenidate (Ritalin), which has a paradoxical calming effect on hyperactive children but a stimulating effect on adults; dextroamphetamine (Dexedrine), the drug you may have taken to stay awake for exams; and pemoline (Cylert), a drug producing a similar alerting effect. These drugs make you feel more energized, much like drinking two cups of strong coffee in the morning. If you are taking a strong pain medicine that makes you drowsy, the stimulants work well to reduce the drowsiness.

If you have been subject to mood swings in the past or have been diagnosed with depression or bipolar disorder, the symptoms may return during cancer treatments. Be sure to continue taking any medications you have been on and tell the oncologist what they are. These are likely to be one or more of the mood stabilizers: lithium (Eskalith), gabapentin (Neurontin), carbamazepine (Tegretol), or divalproex (Depakote). If you have discontinued the one you were taking, it is important to go back to your doctor and discuss whether you should begin taking it again.

OBSESSIVE-COMPULSIVE DISORDER

Obsessive-compulsive disorder (OCD) is characterized by excessive fears, repetitive thoughts, and a need to repeat over and over some action or ritual, like hand washing. If you have a problem in this area, it may complicate the cancer treatment by causing you difficulty in making treatment decisions, inability to undertake or complete a cancer treatment, or worries about accepting a psychotropic drug to treat the obsessive-compulsive disorder. You are likely to be bright and high functioning, and to expect a lot of yourself. You know the fears are irrational, but somehow you can't control them. Fortunately, present-day drugs are highly effective in treating this condition: fluvoxamine (Luvox), fluoxetine (Prozac), paroxetine (Paxil), and clomipramine (Anafranil).

Juanita, forty-five, had suffered from OCD symptoms since early in her adult life. For years, she had an irrational fear of germs that led her repeatedly to wash anything she touched in the kitchen and to wash her hands many times a day. When she shopped, she hesitated to touch objects that had been handled by others.

When a discharge from her right breast developed, Juanita panicked, but told no one. She could not even bring herself to call her doctor. The discharge became worse, and when her family found out, they insisted that she see a doctor. He confirmed a diagnosis of breast cancer. Juanita had a great deal of trouble agreeing to have a mastectomy. She would make up her mind to go through with it, only to panic and feel she couldn't. This occurred twice, and her oncologist became concerned that the time lost was becoming problematic and referred her for help.

Juanita described how her emotional problems had limited her activities over the years. She had attempted psychotherapy once but had refused to consider medication out of fear of the effect a drug might have on her. I proposed that she try paroxetine (Paxil) to lift her depressed and hopeless feelings and reduce her obsessive worrying. After several weeks, her mood lightened; she made an appointment with the doctor and decided to have the surgery.

The routine of the hospital was hard for Juanita, but the staff understood her fears and gave her extra time and attention. The surgery went well, and an early carcinoma was removed. She has continued taking Paxil and has been less limited by her fears.

CONFUSION AND DELIRIUM

One of the most frightening things you can experience during your cancer treatment is having your mind "play tricks" on you. This may be due to one of the medications used to treat the cancer or to treat pain, or it may be due to poor kidney, liver, brain, or lung function. It usually develops not at home, but in the hospital, where the stronger doses of medicines are given and where you are staying if you have significantly impaired function. Opioids, such as morphine for pain, and steroids, such as dexamethasone (Decadron) and prednisone, are the most common drug offenders. If you are taking one of these and experience strange sensations, like misidentifying people or being confused as to what is happening around you, they are likely a side effect of the drug. Sometimes you can get visual hallucinations or feel confused about where you are. Lowering the dose or stopping the drug is usually effective, but a medication may be needed to control the confusion.

Confusion and delirium are reduced by haloperidol (Haldol), thioridazine (Mellaril), olanzapine (Zyprexa), and risperidone (Risperdal). If restlessness or agitation occurs, lorazepam (Ativan) is added.

Table 3 gives the commonly prescribed psychotropic drugs used for patients with cancer. Your oncologist may prescribe one of these or suggest a consultation with a psychiatrist, who will choose the most appropriate drug for you. There must always be communication between the oncologist and psychiatrist to ensure that your medical and psychological care are integrated and that your medication is being monitored so that side effects, if they occur, are recognized. If there are side effects, you and your doctor can decide if and when to stop the drug.

You may have heard of St. John's wort, which is the extract of a plant from Europe that acts as a mild antidepressant. It is being tested further in the United States. St. John's wort generally seems to have no side effects. (In rare cases, however, photophobia, or sensitivity to sunlight, has been reported.) Another "natural" supplement currently used to treat depression is SAM-e (S-adenosyl-methionine), which is produced in the body. It is derived from adenosine triphosphate, which is found in protein-rich food, and has been found to affect depressed mood in adequate doses. Both of these products are available in health food stores. You should tell your oncologist if you take (or are considering taking) St. John's wort, SAM-e, or any other herbs or supplements (see Chapter 10).

In summary, medications are available to ease the psychological symptoms associated with cancer: insomnia, anxiety and panic disorder, depression, fatigue, phobias, obsessive symptoms, and confusion. Psychiatrists and oncologists can choose from a range of available drugs, which, when taken under their supervision, are safe and efficacious. Coping with the day-to-day burdens of cancer becomes tolerable when severe psychiatric symptoms are reduced. Once these symptoms are controlled, your own coping skills can kick in. Table 4 outlines ways to seek help from mental health professionals who are skilled in the psychological problems that commonly complicate cancer care.

TABLE 3

MEDICATIONS COMMONLY USED FOR DISTRESS

	NAMES	
	BRAND	**GENERIC**
SLEEP PROBLEM	Restoril	temazepam
	Ambien	zolpidem
	Klonopin	clonazepam
	Remeron	mirtazapine
	Desyrel	trazodone
	Sonata	zaleplon
ANXIETY/PANIC	Ativan	lorazepam
	Buspar (anxiety only)	buspirone
	Klonopin	clonazepam
	Valium	diazepam
	Librium	chlordiazepoxide
	Xanax	alprazolam
DEPRESSION	Prozac	fluoxetine
	Paxil	paroxetine
	Zoloft	sertraline
	Effexor	venlafaxine
	Serzone	nefazodone
	Celexa	citalopram
	Desyrel	trazodone
	Elavil	amitriptyline
	Wellbutrin	bupropion
	Norpramin	desipramine
	Pamelor	nortriptyline
	Tofranil	imipramine
	Remeron	mirtazapine

	NAMES	
	BRAND	**GENERIC**
MOOD DISORDERS	Tegretol	carbamazepine
	Eskalith	lithium carbonate
	Depakote	divalproex
DEPRESSION AND FATIGUE	Dexedrine	dextroamphetamine
	Ritalin	methylphenidate
	Cylert	pemoline
CONFUSIONAL STATES	Haldol	haloperidol
	Prolixin	fluphenazine
	Zyprexa	olanzapine
	Risperdal	risperidone
	Mellaril	thioridazine
	Thorazine	chlorpromazine
OBSESSIVE-COMPULSIVE DISORDER	Luvox	fluvoxamine
	Anafranil	clomipramine
	Prozac	fluoxetine
	Paxil	paroxetine

TABLE 4

WAYS TO GET HELP

✓ The Resources section of this book provides an extensive list of general organizations and those that deal with specific cancers.

✓ Call 1-800-4 CANCER, the number for information from the National Cancer Institute. Also, call 1-800-ACS-2345 to reach the American Cancer Society Call Line, where bilingual oncology nurses answer questions in English and Spanish twenty-four hours a day. They can recommend resources for help in your community.

✓ Ask your doctor or the oncology nurse or social worker for a referral to a mental health professional or cancer support group.

✓ Ask friends or relatives who have had cancer if they know of a therapist or group that might be right for you.

✓ Ask the advice of a chaplain at the hospital or clergy member from your faith.

✓ Contact your local chapter of organizations such as the American Cancer Society, the Leukemia Society of America, the Wellness Community, or Gilda's Clubs and ask about support services in your area.

ALTERNATIVE AND COMPLEMENTARY THERAPIES

My doctor removed the lobe of my lung that had cancer in it. He told me that was all the treatment I needed. So I started my own treatment program: exercise, Chinese herbs, green tea, vitamin-mineral supplements, and meditation. I just can't stand around and do nothing when my life is at stake.

—Bill, a lung cancer survivor

I feel so much better now that I'm doing something—not just relying on what the doctor can do.

—Laura, a melonoma survivor

I've always believed in the mind-body connection. It has become more important to me now than ever before. I do daily meditation, tai chi, and yoga. I've become more spiritual; I pray every day. All of this gives me a great feeling that I'm using my own resources to help. And I feel in control of my body through my mind.

—Louise, after diagnosis of lymphoma

I've had a pain in my mastectomy scar for three years, which they say is due to a nerve that was cut during surgery. While I understand there's no cure for it, meditation and acupuncture have really helped.

—Nora, a breast cancer survivor

*I feel overwhelmed by all the information I get from the
Internet, friends—everybody—telling me about something
that's really good for my cancer. How do I know what is
credible and what is hype? There's no good way of knowing.*

—John, a man with sarcoma of the right leg

As soon as you heard you had cancer and told a few friends, you
likely began to get calls from them saying, "I just found this new
treatment for your cancer on the Web, and I wanted to be sure you
knew about it. It's supposed to cure your type of cancer and doesn't
harm your body." These calls come at the time you're just trying to
absorb what the doctor has told you about your options for the
conventional medical treatment of your cancer. So now, in addition to the traditional treatments, you have to factor into your
decision the alternative or complementary treatments.

DEFINITION OF ALTERNATIVE AND COMPLEMENTARY THERAPIES

You hear the words *alternative* and *complementary* used loosely and
interchangeably, but you need to know what differentiates them.
The National Institutes of Health has established a National Center
for Complementary and Alternative Medicine, giving us a basis for
understanding the meaning of each term, which is especially important in dealing with cancer. An *alternative* cancer therapy is one that
is promoted as a treatment or cure for cancer, to be used alone,
instead of a conventional cancer treatment. A *complementary* therapy
is one that is not proposed as a cure or treatment for cancer but is
promoted to be used as an adjunct to conventional treatment to help
control symptoms and enhance quality of life. Thus, it is the *purpose*
for which a therapy is used that determines whether it is an alternative or complementary therapy. However, this neat differentiation
becomes blurred in the real world, since most therapies can fall into
either group, depending on how they are used.

For example, in the 1970s guided imagery (visualizing your body's immune system killing the cancer cells) was proposed as a mind-body treatment that could by itself treat cancer, as an alternative therapy. On the other hand, guided imagery with relaxation is widely used nowadays as a complementary therapy, along with conventional cancer treatment; it is a proven and well-accepted method of enhancing the sense of calm and well-being (see Chapter 9). Most people say that "it helps me feel better and it just might help fight the cancer." They do not rely on it as their only cancer treatment but believe that it "might help and won't hurt." This is a way of straddling the fence between alternative and complementary approaches. If you are a strong proponent of mind-body methods, you may find guided imagery helpful as a way for you to assert a sense of control over your illness and its treatment. If you are not a strong believer in the mind-body connection, you will likely use guided imagery as a technique to reduce distress, if you use it at all.

You often see and hear the alternative therapies presented as "natural and nontoxic," in sharp contrast to the side effects you're told about for radiation, chemotherapy, or a formidable surgical procedure. Well, to whom do you listen? What do you do? You're standing at the crossroads: One road leads you to the familiar, mainstream medicine; the other leads you to the panoply of alternative cancer treatments that have become increasingly visible and popular today. Surveys in the United States show that at the present time only about 8 to 10 percent of people will take the alternative route alone and refuse conventional cancer treatment. By far the majority of people with cancer (about 85 percent) go the conventional treatment route and, at the same time, add some of the complementary, trying to get the best of both worlds. They feel, "I'm getting the best treatment for my cancer that medicine has to offer and I might as well explore whatever won't hurt me and just might help." I'm reminded of one of Yogi Berra's comments: "When you get to a fork in the road, take it!" That comes close to describing how many people are dealing with conventional versus alternative modalities: At the fork in the road to cancer therapies, they take both paths.

Alternative and complementary therapies now constitute a billion-dollar industry. Reliable information about them is sometimes hard to find, but much unreliable information is easy to find on thousands of websites. Many of the sites are thinly veiled promotionals or actual advertisements for a particular product. (See Resources at the end of the book for sources of reliable information.) Vitamins, minerals, and food supplements do not come under government regulation; therefore, claims abound that sound too good to be true—and they are likely to be just that! The lack of quality control in their manufacture means that some may be not only ineffective but potentially dangerous. It is helpful to approach this matter with some background, which is offered below.

WHAT TREATMENTS ARE ALTERNATIVE OR COMPLEMENTARY TODAY?

A recent trend classifies only surgery, chemotherapy, immunotherapy, and radiation as conventional cancer treatments. Everything else people do for themselves while receiving one of these treatments is classified as a complementary therapy. Hence diet, exercise, prayer, psychotherapy and counseling, support groups, and meditation are all classified as complementary therapies, accounting in part for the 85 to 90 percent of people using complementary therapies. It seems ridiculous to call psychological support, counseling, and psychotherapy, the use of which is firmly based on research, complementary therapies. It may seem even more absurd to label prayer as a complementary therapy; prayer is a spiritual or religious practice that many people consider a major source of comfort and support whether in good health or in illness. Barrie Cassileth, a sociologist and well-known researcher in alternative and complementary therapies and Chief of the Integrative Medicine Service at Memorial Sloan-Kettering Cancer Center, pointed out:

> *Lifestyle activities, personal care of one's own aches and pain, weight loss programs, and the like do not constitute alternative or complementary activities. They represent living sensibly and taking appropriate responsibility for oneself.*

Currently there is a blurring of the boundary between mainstream and complementary/alternative approaches. Narrowing the gap between the two has helped in ensuring that a potentially useful alternative therapy is recognized and put into a clinical trial to see if it truly is effective. When it proves effective, the alternative therapy joins the ranks of conventional therapies and can be reliably supported for general use. The narrowed gap has also surely helped people who, in the past, had to keep secret from their oncologist their interest in seeking alternative therapies. With more openness in the doctor-patient dialogue, people have been able to talk frankly with their doctors about these ideas. It is important, if you are taking or considering an alternative therapy, to discuss it with your oncologist, because some of these treatments can affect your conventional treatment and should not be used while you are receiving chemotherapy or radiotherapy, particularly anything containing antioxidants. Dr. Cassileth is establishing a useful clearinghouse at Memorial Hospital, where doctors and patients can obtain information on alternative and complementary therapies, including their benefits and risks. Her *Alternative Medicine Handbook* is also helpful (see Resources).

The National Center for Complementary and Alternative Medicine classifies these therapies into seven general categories. Although some have been promoted as alternative treatments for cancer, none at present have been proved effective as a cancer treatment. Trials of the promising ones are in progress. The seven categories are as follows:

Diet and nutrition
Bioelectromagnetics (magnetic fields)
Alternative medicine systems
Pharmacologic and biological therapies
Manual healing
Herbal medicines
Mind-body techniques

The category of diet and nutrition encompasses the megavitamin approaches, metabolic therapies, and the macrobiotic diet, which is based on ancient Chinese ideas of the balance between yin and yang. Bioelectromagnetic approaches relate to the magnetic

field said to exist around the body. Magnets are not a cancer treatment, but they are proving helpful when applied for chronic pain.
Among the alternative medical systems, the most widely used in
cancer treatment are ancient Chinese therapies (traditional Chinese
medicine) using herbs and acupuncture, Ayurvedic medicine from
India, and homeopathy. Pharmacologic and biological therapies of
note include the highly controversial Burzynski's antineoplastons,
Burton's "immunoaugmentive" therapy, and shark cartilage. Several
clinical trials are going on to provide needed information about
these. As yet, none has proved its efficacy as a treatment for cancer.
There are a range of herbal treatments (for example, Essiac and
Hoxsey) that are proposed for cancer. Manual healing involves making use of one's energy field. One form, called therapeutic touch, is
widely used by nurses as a complementary therapy.

Chapter 9 outlines the wide range of types of counseling and
mind-body techniques (such as meditation and relaxation) that are
available to help you cope with cancer today. Many have proved to
be safe and helpful. Although they are all excellent and effective,
none can be proposed as an actual treatment for cancer. Because we
all want to believe that we can have control over our body and illness, these methods have a strong appeal.

Following is a list of some complementary therapies that enhance
well-being and may improve your quality of life:

Acupuncture. Be sure to use a licensed, trained acupuncturist.

Acupressure. Pressing inside the wrist with the fingers
   of the other hand about one inch above the hand
   crease reduces nausea and distress.

Aromatherapy. Fragrances are used for their calming
   effects.

Therapeutic massage. This includes shiatsu, Swedish
   massage, and reflexology (massaging the acupuncture points on the feet.)

Energy healing. Some cancer centers offer Reiki, an "energy healing" technique that originated in Japan and induces deep relaxation.

Yoga. This system incorporates gentle stretching, physical postures, and meditation to induce relaxation and reduce muscle tension.

Ginger root tea. Drinking this tea reduces nausea and coughing.

Tai chi. These gentle Chinese exercises improve well-being and balance.

WHY DO PEOPLE USE COMPLEMENTARY THERAPIES TODAY?

The reasons people add a complementary therapy to their cancer treatment speak to the benefits they attribute to their use:

"I feel more in control."

"I want to be sure I've turned every stone."

"I feel stronger by drawing on the resources of my mind."

"I have to please my family."

"I want to build up my immunity to fight the cancer."

"I am so distressed that I need to calm my fears."

"I want to use everything I can to kill tumor cells."

A more worrisome reason for seeking complementary therapy is the feeling that you aren't getting help for your distress from your oncologist and the conventional medical team, leading to the decision to look for help elsewhere. The *New England Journal of Medicine* (June 3, 1999) reported a study at the Dana Farber Cancer Institute in Boston of the use of alternative therapies among women in the year following treatment for breast cancer. The women who used alternative methods were found to be more fearful about the future, were more depressed, had less sexual satisfaction, and had a poorer quality of life. These women were likely having more trouble coping with their treatment. Yet they were not identified by their doctor as needing help to manage their distress and probably sought complementary therapies on their own. One would hope that oncology teams would be sensitive to recognizing distress and refer such patients for counseling as part of their total cancer care. Your psychological support should be an integral part of your cancer care.

Bonnie provides a good example of many people's views today:

Bonnie, a sixty-year-old, active college professor, was hardly prepared to hear that she had multiple myeloma when she consulted her doctor because of a nagging back pain. She reacted with alarm on learning that there was a malignant tumor in one of her vertebrae, but she felt relieved when her hematologist began chemotherapy and assured her that the tumor had responded well to the treatment. As she reflected more on what the doctor said, she realized that this was a serious, but often chronic disease. She would have to find ways to live with it and keep her life together.

Bonnie's back pain improved, and she continued to teach and carry on her activities with friends. However, she talked with her doctor about wanting "to do something myself to put my body in the best shape to fight this myeloma." The doctor was positive about her idea but said if she planned to take herbs or vitamins, he wanted to know which ones, to be sure she wouldn't take something that would "fight with" the drug treatment for the myeloma. Bonnie found a Chinese doctor who gave her weekly acupuncture treatments to help her back pain and allow her to feel calmer, but he was emphatic that it was not a treatment for her cancer.

Bonnie was never a "health nut," but she believed in "taking care of myself." She found a modified macrobiotic diet that focused on increasing vegetables, fiber, and fruits in her diet. It was not extreme; in fact it closely resembled the food pyramid so widely supported today (see Chapter 12). The diet and a walking routine brought her weight down and increased her stamina.

Bonnie joined a support group where she heard a great deal about the full gamut of alternative and complementary therapies. She tried green tea and found not only that it was good to drink, but that it was being tested in regular clinical trials because of its antioxidant properties. Bonnie found that these lifestyle changes gave her a feeling of getting her life "in order." Her well-being improved. She has coped well by adding her own treatments to the chemotherapy.

DO'S AND DON'T'S FOR ALTERNATIVE AND COMPLEMENTARY THERAPIES

1. DON'T take an alternative therapy in place of a conventional treatment. You may be delaying use of a proven, potentially curative treatment.

2. DO use any of the complementary therapies that make you feel better and help you cope.

3. DON'T believe that if you don't choose to use a particular complementary therapy, you are allow-ing your tumor to grow faster.

4. DO discuss with your doctor any alternative or complementary therapy that you are considering

or taking. Some complementary therapies can interfere with chemotherapy and radiation therapy. If your oncologist doesn't ask, be sure to tell him or her what you are taking.

5. DO seek out reliable sources of information about alternative and complementary therapies (see Resources). Don't rely on a single source, no matter how laudatory.

6. DO be aware that many websites are advertising products that are not subject to quality control in their manufacture, and their claims are unregulated. This continues to be a "buyer beware" market.

7. DO think through your reasons for seeking a complementary therapy. If the reason is that you are having trouble coping, consider asking your oncology team for a referral for counseling. You may be able to have psychological support built into your medical care.

8. DO check the credentials and reliability of the complementary therapist you choose. Be sure you have a licensed acupuncturist, for example, who uses sterile needles. Check into the benefits and risks of each therapy.

9. DO use the complementary therapies that make sense to *you*. You may find that what was great for someone else is not helpful to you at all.

10. DO use the complementary therapies as aids to reducing pain, nausea, and other symptoms, for example, ginger root tea for nausea.

Many of today's complementary and alternative therapies suggest a yearning to return to the ancient sources of wisdom, especially the Eastern tradition, which includes a more mystical orientation, in contrast to Western medicine's empirical, objective, and impersonal approach. In the face of uncertainty, people turn to sources of ancient wisdom with the hope that things that have been known for centuries have inherent validity.

People have their strongly held beliefs about the use of alternative and complementary therapies, which parallel their beliefs about the mind-body connection. Disbelievers remain disbelievers, and believers continue to believe, even in the face of studies that disprove a connection. Scientific studies of alternatives will not likely put these differences to rest because of this central fact of human nature, which is another example of how we each are unique in our mix of views. Even if science does validate an alternative or complementary approach as being helpful in cancer treatment, the research process takes many years. People with cancer become frustrated with this scientific method. They often say, "Dr. Holland, I don't have time to wait for scientific proof. I need to do something now."

In the face of these different points of view, communication remains the key. Many a patient has said to me, "I just believe it works, and that's good enough for me." And that's good enough for me, too, when what they are doing isn't harmful, and they are also getting their regular cancer treatment. Using whatever "it" is fits comfortably into their belief system, and because it does, it offers hope and contributes to the quality of their lives, as well as to their confidence in a good outcome to treatment.

11

"I'M A SURVIVOR—
NOW WHAT?"

*When I got cancer, I asked God to give me two years.
Now that I'm a two-year survivor, I've decided to ask
for more time.*

—Bernadette, a fifty-year-old executive
with uterine cancer

Did *I have cancer? Or do I have cancer?*

—Brooke, a fifty-six-year-old woman who completed
treatment for breast cancer four years earlier,
asking one of the questions most frequently
raised by survivors of cancer

*The doctor quoted statistics to me about my chances for
survival, but I'm not a statistic, I'm me!*

—John, twenty-nine, a three-year survivor
of testicular cancer

*I got a pain the other day in my right earlobe, and I
thought, "My God, it's come back in my right earlobe," knowing how ridiculous that was.*

—Frank, forty-eight, a ten-year survivor of lymphoma

*I used to hate birthdays. Now I'm delighted to celebrate
them.*

—Patrick, a thirty-five-year-old thyroid cancer survivor, who completed treatment two years ago

Breast cancer has become only a piece of the quilt that is my life. I needed to be finished with it, to put a border around the experience. Inside that border are patterns that are familiar to my life, some interesting, some less appealing, and all the flaws that contributed to the creation of the piece. In looking at the piece as a part of the whole quilt, I can view it from different angles, in different light, in relation to all the other pieces. My present task is to take the broader view, to regain a sense of the fullness of my life. . . . The hard task for me and my family is to integrate each of our experiences of cancer into who we are.

—Kathlyn Conway, *Ordinary Life:*
A Memoir of Illness

Kathlyn Conway, a psychotherapist, developed lymphoma as a graduate student, and breast cancer in her early forties. Married with two young children, she wrote a remarkably honest story, *Ordinary Life*, of her reactions to having a mastectomy and chemotherapy. The book details her anger, her depression, and the feeling of having lost her "ordinary life." Written day by day, it describes the daily hassles and stresses of carrying on with her family's life turned upside-down. The stress was hard for her husband, who became fatigued, sometimes despairing, trying to support her while taking care of the children and working at his job. Kathlyn was shocked when she read her diary, written a year earlier during her illness.

Certainly, I set out to write the truth about my cancer while I was still in its grip. I was passionate in my resistance to telling the story that other people seemed to want to hear—of lessons learned, of cancer as a transformative experience. But having told my story, I now find myself startled by its fierceness, its raw and unrelenting character. I almost wish, when I read it over, that it had left me with more of a feeling of transformation.

When the experience of cancer and its treatment is over, it is easy to "rewrite history" and think of yourself as having been more wise, mature, and adaptive than indeed was the case. As with childbirth and other traumas, in retelling it you tend to color the experience as you want to remember it and tell it to others in more acceptable terms. In fact, Kathlyn Conway said, "I doubt that I could write this book today [nineteen months later]. I no longer feel as raw as I did then."

Just as history books are written with the specific slant of the particular historian, so it goes with personal stories of illness. An account written as a daily diary is likely to be the most honest. And over time, some transformative ideas stay with survivors, some good and some "troublesome." These notions are so common, you could almost call them universals (although absolutes about anything are lacking, especially in relation to human emotions).

Brooke, quoted earlier, had a mastectomy at fifty-six, followed by adjuvant chemotherapy (meaning that it was given as part of the initial treatment) for early breast cancer. She continued to work as an interior designer during the chemotherapy, despite being tired. She initially had a hard time adjusting to her "new body" and joined a support group for breast cancer patients and survivors. She found it helpful hearing others describe how they got past the hair loss and adjusted to wearing a wig. She began an exercise and diet routine to keep her weight stable, since women gain weight during chemotherapy and find this an additional problem to deal with. Though she hardly wore makeup at all before her bout with cancer, members of her group suggested she wear more makeup and brighter clothes, both to keep up her spirits and to give her pale look more color. Her husband was very supportive throughout her treatment for cancer, and they both felt that they became closer because of the experience.

At the end of a year, Brooke's appearance and energy level had returned to normal, but her psyche had not. As the time approached for the landmark one-year follow-up visit to her doctor, Brooke came to see me because she recognized that she had suddenly become anxious and irritable and was sleeping poorly. She said, "I feel well, and I usually don't worry about my health. But when the flu was going around my office, and I started feeling achy all over, I thought, 'What if it's *not* the flu? What if the cancer's come back?' I worked myself into a real panic. Then I started wondering, 'What if they didn't really get it all? What if I'm *not* cured?' My husband tells me it's all in my head. There's nothing wrong with me, and I'm just obsessing. He says, 'You beat it. Be grateful, and move on.' But I'm not so sure. I called my doctor, and she said it was nearly time for my next checkup so why didn't I just come in *now*? I scheduled an appointment for next week, and I haven't been able to sleep ever since. All I can think of is: What if they find something?" She took a deep breath and said, "The crazy part of this is: I feel fine. My life is great. I'm just so terrified that at any moment I could lose it all."

Brooke's story exemplifies the phenomenon my colleagues and I described years ago when we followed women through their treatment regimen of mastectomy and radiation for breast cancer. We expected women to be jubilant on finishing treatment; in fact, the opposite occurred. They had a paradoxical *increase* in distress just after treatment, and we learned then about this feeling of vulnerability on finishing treatment. Two main factors caused this new and unexpected anxiety: the fear that the cancer could come back now that they were without the protective effects of treatment, and the fear that they were not being watched as closely by their doctors.

Most cancer survivors typically experience what Brooke went through, wondering, "*Did* I have cancer? Or *do* I still have cancer?" Angelo, a thirty-eight-year-old lymphoma survivor, put it this way: "I think I'll never feel as confident about my life, myself, and the future as I did before I had cancer." We call this common feeling in survivors the Damocles syndrome. According to the Greek legend, Damocles, a courtier to the tyrant Dionysius, the Elder of Syracuse, extravagantly praised his sovereign, who invited him to a sumptuous feast. However, during the entertainment, Damocles looked up and saw that Dionysius had seated him directly beneath a sword that was suspended from the ceiling by a thread. For Damocles, this sword was a symbol of the precariousness of life and how one's fortune could shift from being in favor at court to falling out of favor, causing the sword to fall down on one's head. For people who have had cancer, that sword represents the frailty and precarious nature of life itself. They continue to believe that the threat of recurring cancer—and consequently, the threat of death—is always looming over them.

Usually, this fear slowly recedes as the time from diagnosis and treatment increases. But the fear exacerbates just before follow-up visits, scans, and tests for cancer. It also may reappear around significant anniversaries related to the cancer, such as the day of the diagnosis or the surgery.

"I can't get the cancer out of my mind. It keeps coming back with the silliest reminders," said Martina, a young woman who survived uterine cancer. Rather than silly, these are normal and ubiquitous concerns; unfortunately, they "go with the territory." They, too, get better over time. I often use a novel approach in dealing with these fears, which I learned from Dr. Christopher Gates, a psychiatrist colleague. He helps the person to conceptualize these fears by saying:

> Just imagine with me that your frightening thoughts are like voices on a radio. They can be controlled by changing the volume. When the volume is up too high, the noise (your fear) is so loud you can't hear or think of anything else. But you can turn the volume down, so low that you still hear the noise (your fear) in the background, but it doesn't bother you so much, and you can concentrate on other things.

This "mind-gimmick" is helpful since it also implies that those "gremlins" are always going to be there after cancer. They never *completely* go away, but they can be turned down so they can be tucked into the far corner of your brain where they aren't "noisy."

Even individuals who went through their treatment years ago may still find it frightening, even terrifying, to go to their doctor. Other events may reawaken these fears, such as media coverage of the illness or death from cancer of a prominent figure (see Chapter 6), as when Mickey Mantle and Jacqueline Kennedy Onassis died.

On the other hand, cancer success stories such as that of Tour de France cycling champion Lance Armstrong, a testicular cancer survivor, can inspire and give hope to people with cancer and their families.

It's best to approach predictable, anxiety-provoking periods by talking about them with others: family, friends, support group members, or a psychotherapist or counselor, if the anxiety interferes with normal activities. It is helpful mentally to "count to ten" and recall, rationally, that your tests have been negative, you feel fine, and the fears are coming from an external stimulus. Severe and persistent fears (discussed in Chapter 6), however, should prompt a consultation with a mental health professional, with whom you can try some relaxation techniques. If antianxiety medication is needed, consultation with a psychiatrist will be helpful.

AM I A CANCER PATIENT OR A CANCER SURVIVOR?

There is a lot of debate about who qualifies as a cancer survivor. Researchers who study long-term effects of treatments define a survivor as a person who completed treatment at least five years ago and has no sign of cancer. But the National Coalition for Cancer Survivorship (NCCS), an advocacy group composed of cancer survivors, says that a far better way to define *survivor* is to assume that one is a survivor from the day of diagnosis. I find this much more helpful. Dr. Fitzhugh Mullen, the physician and cancer survivor who established the NCCS, says, using this definition, that there surely are different "seasons of survival," but each has to do with survival. The first season is surviving the treatment; the second season is beginning to return to normal life; and the third is the long-term adjustment during which the cancer comes to be viewed as an episode in the bigger context of one's life.

My colleagues and I have become increasingly concerned about the human side of survival from cancer. What "psychological baggage" do you carry around with you? What are your worries about the possible long-term medical problems? What happens to family relations? How does having had cancer affect your perspective on life and its meaning? What happens to your sense of the future? What happens to your ability to become close and intimate with someone? Is it safe to plan a marriage and have children? This baggage is the downside of the remarkably good news that there are, today, nearly eight million cancer survivors, as more cancers respond to new therapies.

The questions we have been studying about the human side of survivorship can be placed under the larger topic of "quality-of-life" issues: How well are you able to function in physical, psychological, social, work, and sexual terms, compared with how you functioned before your illness? One of the breakthroughs concerning the human side of cancer has been the ability to measure and put realistic numbers on a person's functioning in these domains of living, which represent, collectively, quality of life. Nowadays, when we test a new treatment for cancer against an older one to determine which of the two treatments is better, we not only look at *how much longer* people survive with each treatment, but also determine *how well* have they survived (their quality of life) during that time (see Chapter 7).

This interest in the quality of life also extends to our study of survivors. In fact, the National Cancer Institute established an Office of Cancer Survivorship in 1997 to give proper attention to this area.

My twenty years of working in cancer medicine has seen a 180-degree change in attitudes about survivors. When cancer was almost uniformly fatal, a survivor was so rare that any complaint by the patient was countered with "You should just be thankful you're alive." The focus of the oncologists then was to reverse the balance that most often resulted in death and make it possible to become a survivor. They had little time to delve into the problems that the few survivors had, like trouble getting a job because the assumption was they would die, sexual problems, or problems adjusting to physical losses, like a limb or a breast.

The picture started changing in the 1950s and 1960s, when a remarkable increase in survival from several tumors of children and young adults occurred. Suddenly, children with acute lymphocytic leukemia were being put in remission and remained so years later following combination chemotherapy (several drugs given together). Between the mid-1960s and now, the five-year survival rate for Hodgkin's disease rose from 5 percent to greater than 90 percent for Stage I disease, owing to the use of radiotherapy and combination chemotherapy regimen (called MOPP, for the names of the drugs used). Testicular cancer became largely curable in young men. With these changes came a new concern, one that had not been possible before: What were the problems, the downside, associated with the treatments, and how could they be reduced? For example, early treatments for childhood leukemia included radiation to the brain to prevent the leukemia cells from being sequestered there only to regrow at a later time, but it caused some children to have trouble with learning and performance at school. Could the radiation be eliminated and still effect a cure in the children? This has indeed happened.

Chemotherapy for Hodgkin's disease caused infertility. Could every young man with Hodgkin's be asked to bank sperm, and could a regimen be found that did not cause infertility? Both changes have occurred: Teenage boys and men with Hodgkin's disease can bank sperm before undergoing high-dose chemotherapy. And the Hodgkin's disease MOPP regimen, which caused sterility most of the time, has been replaced by the ABVD regimen, which is as effective but does not cause sterility.

For the first time, the focus of medical efforts was on survivors: keeping the cure rates high, while reducing the negative impacts of treatments. It was in this exciting period of change in the 1970s that interest in psychological issues developed and that my group was established at Memorial. It was a new era of concern for the human side of cancer.

THE TYRANNY OF STATISTICS

One of the burdens cancer survivors often carry is information about the statistics for survival for their particular cancer. The question so often asked by a person who receives the diagnosis of cancer is, "What are my chances, Doc?" No matter what the answer is, anything less than 100 percent survival (which is, of course, what everyone wants to hear) leads to the nagging fear of "which group am I going to be in, the 50 percent who make it or the 50 percent who don't?"

The numbers that a doctor gives you are based on the expected average survival at a particular time, often five years. The trouble with statistics is that no one person is the exact "average." So the numbers become another monkey on your back, an added fear to deal with. Doctors want to be honest and sometimes give the range from the shortest to the longest likely survival; they tell you truthfully they can't predict exactly where you will fall.

In dealing with statistics, I'm often reminded of the stranger who pulled into a little town in the Ozarks. The stranger saw an old man sitting outside the country store and yelled, "Old-timer, can you tell me what the death rate is around these parts?" The old man looked at him and said, "I reckon it's still one per person." The point is that you can't take the quoted average survival time too gloomily. It's an average and, as John said, as quoted at the beginning of this chapter, "I'm not a statistic, I'm me."

It's helpful to talk with survivors who, twenty years later, can describe the dire "you have six months to live" prognosis they were given. They understand the burden of the statistics they were saddled with. Many of these people have donated their time and energy to making sure that other cancer patients get good information, good support, and good treatment.

Natalie Spingarn was one such twenty-year-plus survivor of metastatic breast cancer. She was a writer in Washington, D.C., and the author of *The New Cancer Survivors,* which is an excellent book on the human side of cancer (see Resources). She was a founding member of the National Coalition for Cancer Survivorship (NCCS), writing and speaking often as an advocate for patients.

Richard Block, founder with his brother of the H & R Block firm for tax preparation assistance, is a survivor of lung cancer of twenty-plus years. He was told, "Go home and write your will; there is no treatment for your problem." He refused to accept that verdict and, with his wife, Annette, sought out the best cancer centers. He was treated and is healthy and working hard to ensure that patients with cancer get accurate information. He and Annette established a center in Kansas City where patients are seen by consultants in surgery, oncology, and radiotherapy. Several years ago, he gave the National Cancer Institute the funds to start a service to provide updated information to patients on which centers have protocols to treat specific tumors. The result was the 1-800-4-CANCER telephone number, which is accessible, in user-friendly language, to anyone. He and Annette have written about their experiences and are ardent activists. Richard feels keeping hope alive is a critical part of the human side of cancer.

Bob Fisher was an inspiration to me and my group. He was treated at our hospital for chronic myelocytic leukemia. For eight years, he worked as a volunteer with us, counseling newly diagnosed leukemia patients. He taught us much about what a volunteer can do to help patients. His initial work provided the spark for a program developed at Memorial Hospital called the Patient-to-Patient Volunteer Program, which provides a patient counselor for the range of tumors commonly seen. The program now has over twenty-five survivors of more than twenty different types of cancer. These volunteers are from all walks of life, corporate executives to blue-collar workers, and they come to the hospital to talk with patients who have the same type of cancer that they had.

This organization provides yet another example of survivors who want to "give back" by helping new patients, and both benefit. Volunteers act as "buddies" or guides, who speak with the authority of having "been there." Consequently, they share their experiences and offer their tried-and-true advice on coping as well as practical tips, such as where to shop for wigs and prostheses, how to get ostomy appliances, and how to deal with fatigue and worry.

And they offer that "gift of hope," by their very presence, as a survivor of the same cancer.

In a lecture at the Joan and Sanford I. Weil Medical College of Cornell University, Susan Sontag, author of *Illness as Metaphor*, spoke about how her experience with breast cancer, twenty-four years ago, led her to write this important book. She was given a pessimistic prognosis but pursued aggressive treatment and is alive these many years later. She felt that the prevalence of cancer as a metaphor for bad things in society made the burden of cancer even greater for patients and survivors. Her writing and public speaking about her experience give testimony to the fact that statistics about prognoses can be pretty meaningless. She also decries the idea that personality could be the cause of cancer—or the cure. Cancer is just another disease and is better left free of such implications, she believes. The bottom line is that statistics are just statistics. Prognoses are based on "ballpark" averages and should be kept in perspective, because each of us is unique.

The question asked earlier in the chapter by Brooke, "Am I cured?" is the biggest question for most survivors. Of course, everyone wants to hear the answer "yes!" It's interesting that in earlier days you were more likely to get that answer. After mastectomy, surgeons would tell their patients, "You're cured. Come back to see me in a year." Today, the pendulum has swung the other way. Few oncologists I know are comfortable telling their patients they are cured, because it implies an absolute certainty that is anathema to these scientifically trained clinicians. They prefer terms like "likely cured" or "no evidence of disease" or "long-term remission." This approach often frustrates and angers patients, who want a sure answer. Here is one of those instances in which the profound uncertainty of living with cancer is deeply felt, and the doctor's words don't always reassure. The desired assurance is withheld in the service of not promising something one isn't sure about. Hope, that sustaining feeling, is muted by the caution of doctors.

Cancer survivors usually have follow-up visits scheduled every three months for the first year after treatment ends and every six months thereafter, depending on the tumor. This sometimes creates the impression that the cancer is lurking about and the doctor is expecting it to reappear. There has been some debate as to whether survivors are followed at too frequent intervals. Given present knowledge, however, it is better to know early if the tumor has come back, so that something can be done. Consequently, we are caught in the vise of sacrificing the sense of security that would come with less frequent follow-up for the repeated anxiety that precedes the more frequent follow-ups, which usually net negative results, but that *would* pick up early recurrence. We are left with finding ways to control the anxiety that accompanies the checkups.

PHYSICAL PROBLEMS OF SURVIVAL: THE DOWNSIDE OF TREATMENTS

Some cancer treatments produce few long-term, physical side-effects, whereas others take a toll on your ability to function normally. These side effects, of course, add to the psychological burden, based on what they are and what function they impair. These visible signs of cancer, with which people live out their lives, create a stigma: People perceive these survivors as "different."

Dr. Alice Kornblith, a research psychologist who has studied survivors, uses the concept of stigma proposed by sociologist Dr. Erving Goffman. He noted that the more people are obviously different from others, the greater is the potential for them to be stigmatized and isolated. The operations that produce visible changes in appearance and permanent disability lead to more stigma: limb amputation; mastectomy; surgery around the face and head; loss of the voice box; colostomy.

Radiation and chemotherapy usually cause less obvious and visible changes, but these treatments may result in impaired function. For example, some chemotherapy regimens can result in damage to the brain, liver, or kidneys, as well as to sexual and reproductive function for both men and women, causing long-term problems. As vexing as these problems can be, they are sometimes the unfortunate downside of the treatments that make it possible to *be* a survivor.

A potential and devastating effect of both radiation and chemotherapy is that they can, years later, result in second tumors. This explains the great interest in and increasing research into long-term treatment effects, especially in childhood survivors, who can expect to live out a full life span. The Children's Cancer Group, a large cooperative group composed of most academic pediatric oncologists in the United States, is currently studying about twenty thousand children treated by protocols over the past decade. They will follow these survivors carefully to look for the factors associated with impaired function or second malignancies and impaired quality of life. This research will be the basis for altering treatment regimens to maintain the gains in survival but reduce the risk of future harm.

Karen Swymer is an inspiring cancer survivor who was diagnosed with Ewing's sarcoma in the right forearm in 1980, the day before her eleventh birthday. Here is her story in her own words:

My consciousness began on June 30, 1980. The doctors asked if I ever had measles, chickenpox . . . then they told me what I did have. My mother looked at me and said, "If I could do this for you I would." And then I started chemo the day of diagnosis. After my first chemo, my parents carried me out of the hospital. I felt like a train ran over me.

I had chemo every two and a half weeks. Then I did whatever it took to get back to school on Monday. I wanted to be around kids. I didn't want to interrupt my life. For two weeks we'd soar, and then for a week or so I'd be sick, and we'd cope with it. In those days, there were no medicines to keep you comfortable like there are now. It was like a hell ride because I was so sick. I also had radiation every day for three months over the summer.

I lost my hair for two years, from age eleven to age thirteen. That's a tough time to be bald. People who are in your little circle of friends know you and love you. But if I was out at the movies or the grocery store, people would stare at me. I always held my head up high, but people remind you you're different.

But I had a wonderful little life. I played the flute. I was involved in student government. I was a normal child for all intents and purposes. When I was sick, people were not very open in terms of talking about the disease. Families were very private. People coped very privately, particularly with pediatric cancer. Our family was like a little island. My parents and three sisters were always around me. I was never alone.

After two years, my treatment was over. I went on to high school and then to Smith College. My cancer was behind me. It was something that made me different inside, but looking at me you'd never know. I worked extra hard, played hard, and loved twice as deeply. I loved every part of my life. I clung to my relationships, my future, and my family. I felt invincible. I felt that I'd seen the worst life had given me.

After college, I lived and worked in Washington, D.C., at a public relations firm and then at a law firm. I started having discomfort in the arm where the sarcoma had been. It turned out to be a degenerative condition called necrosis, the dying of the bone. It was the result of the radiation I had received as a child. (When I received it, they were giving a lot more radiation in a larger area than they do now. Over the years, they've learned how much is too much.)

So in the spring of 1993 they found a benign tumor in my elbow. They reconstructed my elbow with part of my hipbone and put some metal hardware in there. I went off to law school in the fall. It was painful but I wasn't worried about being sick.

Eventually it got worse to the point that I could barely hold a pen. They removed the ulna [a bone in the arm] to reduce the chance of my getting sick and reconstructed the entire arm. But two months after starting my second year of law school, I had a malignant tumor in my elbow. It was an osteosarcoma, a different disease. And the cancer had metastasized to both my lungs.

My chemo was more vigorous, with three out of every

five weeks in the hospital and then two weeks off, for a year and a half. It physically beat me down. I had surgery removing the tumors from both lungs. And I lost my right arm.

I was on the pediatric oncology floor even though I was twenty-five years old, to stay with the doctor who had treated me as a child at the Jimmy Fund in Boston. It's very different when your doctor feels like your partner and listens to you and answers you.

I don't think much about losing my arm. It encompasses so little of my time and energy and thought. I've taught myself to write left-handed, and every so often I'll sketch and it makes me feel good. There's nothing I can't do. I just have to be more creative about how I do things. I don't feel limited in any way.

It's a loss. But such an insignificant one to me. Recently, I went to get a key made. I was trying to put my money back in my wallet one-handed. The guy at the store saw me and said, "I'm really sorry about it." And I said, "Worse things can happen."

I have peace of mind and heart that I did whatever it took to get better. Your spiritual presence comes forth and that's how you survive. Physically I looked horrendous, but spiritually you couldn't shake me. If God wanted me to do this every fifteen years, I wouldn't be too happy, but I'd do it because I've had a great life.

Karen Swymer returned to Boston College Law School in 1997 and graduated in 1999. She recently started her first job as an attorney at Sullivan & Worcester, LLP in Boston, Massachusetts. She frequently visits children with cancer in the hospital to give them hope.

The American Cancer Society, under the direction of Dr. Frank Baker, a psychologist, is undertaking a study of fifteen thousand survivors of the major cancers to assess the quality of their lives years after treatment.

It is heartening that research in oncology is now targeting survivors to determine their physical problems, their health, and their quality of life. This is a far cry from the admonition, mentioned earlier, given to survivors twenty-five years ago, not to complain about a thing because "you should just be thankful you are alive."

AFTER TREATMENT: LONG-TERM SURVIVAL

We have talked about the panicky feelings that plague many people when they finish treatment: the paradoxical increase in distress and vulnerability well characterized as the Damocles syndrome. These universals of early survival diminish over time. But in the longer term, how people get along depends on the mix of factors that contribute to how all of us manage: the combination of health, supportive family or friends, philosophical and spiritual resources, basic financial stability, and a satisfactory work life.

GIVING BACK

Often a person who has survived cancer has a desire to "give back" and seeks a way to do it. Sheila Kussner of Montreal is such a remarkable person and a dear friend and coconspirator in the fight to obtain greater resources to fund research for improving psychological care of patients.

At age fourteen, Sheila developed an osteogenic sarcoma, which required the amputation of her leg. Now, years later and a grandmother, she can reflect on what it was like as a teenage girl to wear a prosthetic limb. But Sheila's dynamic personality led her to begin to visit every patient at the Montreal Jewish General Hospital who had an amputation to give that unique, personal support and understanding that only she, a fellow traveler, could give. She has continued that practice through the years.

Sheila married Marvin Kussner, a Montreal businessman, and they have two grown daughters. Sheila's charisma,

energy, enthusiasm, and commitment have resulted in the
raising of millions of dollars for cancer research. Fifteen years
ago, she conceived and established a program at the Montreal
Jewish General Hospital called Hope and Cope. It has grown
and developed into an internationally recognized program
providing psychological support and practical services to
thousands of patients with cancer. Using a large number of
volunteers, many of whom have had cancer or have been
involved in cancer through a relative's illness, the organization
is a powerhouse of caregivers and fundraisers. Bob Fisher, the
leukemia survivor mentioned earlier, and I had the pleasure
of helping in the conception and launching of Hope and
Cope. It is a model program that reflects Sheila's dedication to
the well-being of cancer patients. Through their strong dedication, Sheila and Marvin Kussner have made significant
contributions to the human side of cancer.

Like Sheila, who started to "give back" as a teenage cancer survivor, many cancer survivors gain a sense of meaning and purpose in
doing something for others with cancer. This is a remarkably important way of giving back because seeing and talking with a live human
being who has beat the odds and survived your type of cancer is a
more tangible sign that you, too, can survive than any words of wisdom or encouragement from a doctor. It is truly a gift of hope and
can be given only by someone who has been there. Hope is so
important early on, and a volunteer, by his or her presence, makes a
new patient feel, "If you made it, I can, too."

For the volunteer survivor, the other side of giving back is the
feeling of reward for having helped someone else with the same
problem. In discussions with the Patient-to-Patient Volunteers at
Memorial, my colleagues and I have continually been struck by their
frequently voiced conviction: "We [volunteers] get as much out of it
[the encounter] as they [the patients] do."

This conviction stems from various points of view, including
these:

1. "I wouldn't want anyone else to have to go through what I went through," says Mary, a breast cancer survivor in her sixties who had a mastectomy when such things were rarely discussed and when little support was available.

2. "I kept thinking 'something good' has to come of this," says Frank, a forty-year-old Hodgkin's disease survivor. "I found the opportunity to help other patients is one of the good things that have come out of my cancer—and it's enough for me."

3. "This patient-to-patient volunteering constantly reminds me how strong I am, how much I have endured, and how far I have come," says Lourdes, a sarcoma survivor. "I was just as scared as they are. Helping them gives me a sense of appreciation and gratitude for my own journey."

Jay Weinberg is a twenty-five-year survivor of metastatic melanoma, who was given a poor likelihood of survival. But he has remained well and has devoted his retirement years to helping others with cancer. Jay is not only a founding member of Patient-to-Patient Volunteers but also founder of the Corporate Angels Network (CAN). Jay was concerned that many cancer patients did not have access to the best care because they could not afford the high cost of airfare to get a special treatment that was available only at a particular major cancer center. So he recruited business executives to provide empty seats on their corporate jets. Operating out of the Westchester Airport near New York City, Corporate Angels matches patients who need to be flown to different cities for their cancer treatments with corporations, which donate seats on their corporate jets. For information about contacting the Corporate Angels Network, see Resources at the end of this book.

WORK AND INSURANCE ISSUES

Charlotte, a thirty-eight-year-old saleswoman, completed her chemotherapy treatment for lymphoma one year ago. Since she returned to work, Charlotte says, "Everyone treats me funny. It seems like someone's always telling me 'You look great!' which makes me think either I must have really looked horrible when I was sick or that everybody thinks if you have cancer you're supposed to look like death warmed over, so how come I don't? People ask, 'How are you?' in this very pointed way, as if they're assuming something must be wrong. Or they ask me if I'm too cold from the air conditioning, or something like that. Actually, I'd be fine if people stopped relating to me like some kind of freak."

Arthur, a thirty-year-old leukemia survivor, works as an attorney at a large Wall Street law firm. He says, "I work in a very conservative firm. I got a lot of snide comments about my 'buzz cut' when I came back to work before all my hair had grown back from chemo. Like, 'All you need now is an earring and tattoo.' I just didn't feel like explaining and answering their questions."

Though Arthur was on a fast track for a promotion, he feels that his advancement has been derailed by his illness. "I'm not getting the number or quality of referrals I got before I was sick," he says. "At first, I thought I was getting a cushy workload so I could recover my endurance and not have to work such long hours, which was great when I felt tired a lot. But now that I'm stronger, I feel that I'm not considered able to perform normally. I don't know if people think I'm tainted because I had cancer, or if they think I'm no longer reliable, because they're afraid I might have to go back to the hospital at any moment or I might drop dead. As if the same thing couldn't happen to them.

"But what really gets me is that I can't say anything; I can't rock the boat. If they get upset with me and I eventually lose this job, I'm afraid I wouldn't get another one with my health history. What other employer would take me on knowing I had cancer? And if that happened, how would I get my health insurance? I know how expensive it is to buy on your own. Yeah, it's illegal to discriminate based on medical history, but there are plenty of other reasons they can give for not hiring me."

The work issues extend to parents of childhood survivors. I talked with David, the forty-three-year-old father of five-year-old Michelle, who had acute lymphocytic leukemia a year earlier at Memorial Sloan-Kettering Cancer Center.

Michelle came through her initial treatment well, and all looked hopeful for her. Of course, her parents were grateful and delighted to have Michelle returning to good health. However, the family was covered under David's health insurance plan at his job as a radiology technician. He said, "I have a lot of problems with my supervisor, and I want to change jobs to improve my situation. But how can I risk a gap in my health insurance coverage if I change jobs? I feel I'm 'stuck' in my job. They've been good about giving me time off when Michelle was sick. To be honest, I'm just *afraid* to make a change."

The concern about changing jobs is an important issue for survivors. It calls for revealing the cancer diagnosis with the possibility of job discrimination or difficulty in obtaining new health insurance coverage.

Sometimes realistic issues arise involving physical problems that complicate work:

Lynn is a fifty-four-year-old breast cancer survivor. "I'm a librarian, and one of the simplest things I do every day is take these heavy reference books off the shelf whenever someone wants to look at one. Well, I've never given that part of my job a thought. But since I had the lymph nodes removed from under my right arm as part of my breast surgery, it's really hard for me to lift them. On one hand, I didn't want to strain or hurt my arm because I'm worried about it swelling up [lymphedema]. On the other hand, it seemed silly to ask someone for help every time I needed to grab one of these volumes. They would wonder why I couldn't do it myself. I talked with my boss, who understood my predicament and moved me to another area, where I can use my skills to help people with computer searches. I hated to own up to the fact that I simply couldn't do that part of my job on a long-term basis, but it was a realistic decision, and now things are working out well."

While legislation exists ostensibly to protect people who cannot do their original job, such laws are not always respected. This problem falls harshly on blue-collar workers, whose jobs entail more physical effort. There are resources available when an employer is discriminating in subtle or obvious ways. The National Coalition for Cancer Survivorship (NCCS) and the Center for Patient Advocacy provide opportunities for legal advice. Also, it's possible to appeal a case through state and federal offices. It is wise to get some counsel early concerning your legal rights.

Surveys have shown that the concerns about poor work performance of cancer survivors are myths that need to be dispelled. It is important to remind employers that, overall, about three out of four cancer survivors are able to resume their jobs at the level of employment they held before they were diagnosed with cancer.

The extent of job discrimination is difficult to pinpoint, but large numbers of cancer survivors have reported it, varying from being fired, laid off, or pressured to leave; to being demoted, given less desirable work, or denied a promotion or raise; to having a hard time finding a new job.

The following attitudes and misconceptions about cancer, held by employers or coworkers, have contributed to job discrimination:

1. The old idea of calling cancer a death sentence.
   Therefore, in the long run, people who have been

treated for cancer are considered more of a liability to a company than an asset. They may also raise the cost of insurance for the group.

2. Cancer survivors will be unable to work up to par, either because of more absences, less strength, or less ability to perform.

3. Cancer may be contagious. It may be unsafe to work next to someone who has cancer.

In spite of these misconceptions and biases, nearly two out of three cancer survivors claim that their employers and coworkers have been helpful and supportive to them by modifying work schedules so they could go to medical appointments and by relieving them of taxing physical tasks to accommodate their needs. Indeed, in the United States, the Americans with Disabilities Act (ADA) prohibits employment discrimination based on disability and demands that employers must provide an "accommodation" for a disability; for example, the employer must provide access to the worksite to individuals in wheelchairs. Under this law, it is illegal to discriminate against a worker who can perform a task with a reasonable accommodation. Another law, the Rehabilitation Act of 1973, which applies to employers who receive federal financial assistance, was extended in the 1990s to include cancer survivors. This law prohibits discrimination against people with a medical condition that has no effect on their ability to perform the particular job at hand.

The changes taking place in our society to counter discrimination are all in the right direction, but each situation is different, and the earlier advice to seek counsel about your options is worth repeating here.

Health care is in such flux in the United States that it is difficult to predict whether or not the worries about insurance will be addressed. At present, through federal law, you can retain your health insurance plan for eighteen months if you become unemployed by paying for it yourself. There are moves to prevent higher rates being charged for those with a history of particular illnesses. It is likely that at least some of these problems will be corrected in the next decade. The Center for Patient Advocacy can provide you with information and advice regarding these issues.

FAMILY AND FRIENDS

Chapter 3 describes in detail how important social support and ties (family and friends) are in adapting to cancer. This is no less the case for survivors. In terms of the impact of cancer on marriages of survivors, good marriages get stronger, but marriages that were poor before the onset of cancer are not likely to get better. Studies show, however, that divorce rates are no higher among cancer survivors than among the healthy population. Also, parents of a child with cancer are no less likely to divorce than a couple whose children are healthy. However, when the cancer survivor experiences the loss of a significant other through either conflict, divorce, or death, it adds a burden to coping with long-term cancer issues. Clearly, a stable intimate relationship is helpful to survivors.

There is no question, however, that even the most loving and stable marriages are challenged and stressed when one of the partners has gone through cancer, as Kathlyn Conway described. One of the most common problems is the feeling that the spouse (and nearly everyone else) just has no clue to how the cancer patient feels. I commonly hear the refrain "He [or she] just doesn't understand." Survivors may find their loved ones are overly solicitous and are unable to "put the cancer behind" them when the survivor would like to. Sometimes, survivors feel perfectly fine but are prevented by loved ones from doing anything "strenuous" lest they hurt themselves, which can make the survivor feel overprotected, even humiliated. Changing this pattern without hurting the spouse is hard, especially during the early stages of survival (see Chapter 15).

Similar problems occur for child survivors, whose parents are often hypervigilant in looking for any signs of illness and restricting the child's return to normal behaviors and activities out of fear that their child might "catch something." Family members often ask for help in dealing with these issues. They ask, "How much do I protect or do myself? To what extent should I let go? How much should we talk about cancer? Am I making it worse?"

Sometimes, the opposite response is seen in the spouse or other loved ones: the assumption that the survivor is now well and that medical problems are all over. The survivor is easily fatigued, easily stressed, and yet the healthy spouse doesn't seem to "get it." Both are experiencing battle fatigue that sinks in when the crisis is over; each needs great consideration from the other, yet neither can identify what's wrong. In these instances, couples therapy or family therapy is needed to secure a return to normalcy.

I recall the case of Linda, whose husband, Scott, had been quite physically active all of their married life together:

Throughout their marriage, Linda had depended on Scott to keep the house together, manage repairs, mow the lawn, and be the "mover and shaker" of the family. After hormonal therapy for prostate cancer, Scott was slowed down and could barely take out the garbage. Yet as soon as his treatment was over, Linda expected him to "return to normal." She couldn't get used to his inactivity. Linda felt that pushing Scott would be better than accepting his limited activities, which left him feeling inadequate and depressed. She needed assurance that he was doing all he could so she could accept this level as his best.

Scott eventually became stronger, but I had to sit Linda down and tell it to her straight that he wasn't being lazy, he wasn't faking it. He simply didn't have the energy to take out the garbage, and could she please lay off him and find another way to get the garbage out of the house every night? She was shocked. She said, "But Dr. Holland, I thought he was better." I said, "He *is* better. But he can't take out the garbage."

Many people do regain their ability to perform all or nearly all the tasks they performed before they became ill. But many find, as detailed in Chapter 7, that they need to modify or avoid certain tasks or activities soon after their treatment or, in some cases, permanently.

Other times, we see the Superman or Superwoman syndrome, in which the survivor ignores common sense and tries to prove how strong he or she is. One young wife was appalled when her husband, who recently had surgery for colon cancer, climbed up on the roof of their house to fix the antenna. "He didn't need to prove to me that he's still a real man by risking his life after having surgery a month ago," she said. "He could have been killed after surviving his cancer."

One piece of good news regarding relationships after cancer is that many survivors (about one out of three) report that their cancer has resulted in positive changes in their relationships with their friends. People experienced deeper friendships with really close friends.

Another study found survivors complained that both family and friends, who were devoted during the crisis of the illness, became increasingly *less* supportive as time went on. Some survivors said that this was the "single most distressing hardship of long-term survival." Sometimes, people aren't clear how much to "hover" and how much to go on with "business as usual." Likely, it's best if you, the survivor, give off signals as to what you actually need. We all vary in how much attention we need from others, and in this instance defining that need for others may help.

You may find it hard to talk about continuing problems, both physical and psychological, that are due to cancer. It is important to let the people close to you know that even though you are cancer free, you still have fears and moments of sadness or other emotions related to cancer for which you need support. Some survivors face persistent reminders of their cancer because of a physical loss that continues to require an adjustment. And they are not helped by others saying "you should be used to it by now." Because of these attitudes, the cancer survivor may find it difficult to share how hard it still is or that occasional wave of upset that comes up from time to time. In these instances, a self-help group is a great resource because it's made up of other survivors who have had similar experiences and dealt with similar issues, what Sheila Kussner (introduced earlier in this chapter) calls "sisters under the skin."

POSTTRAUMATIC STRESS DISORDER

Most of the problems with which cancer survivors cope fall into the domain of distress, which would not qualify as a bona fide psychiatric disorder. However, one form of anxiety appears often enough in cancer survivors that it should be mentioned here: posttraumatic stress disorder (PTSD), previously mentioned in Chapter 6.

The term *posttraumatic stress disorder* was popularized by Dr. Lenore Terr, a psychiatrist. She studied twenty-three children who in 1976 were kidnapped at gunpoint while in their schoolbus in Chowchilla, California, and held hostage. They were buried underground in their bus before they escaped. Terr discovered that, some time after this traumatic event, fourteen of the twenty-three children suffered from mental flashbacks of the event, frequently replaying it in their minds. They also had symptoms of increased arousal of the autonomic nervous system, such as being startled by loud noises, high anxiety, difficulty sleeping, poor concentration, nightmares, irritability, and anger. Some Vietnam veterans showed the same symptoms after combat. The disorder has increasingly been described among those who have experienced a frightening, traumatic event, including a natural disaster, rape or physical abuse, or combat.

Professionals have begun to recognize these symptoms in cancer survivors as well. In the first studies, it looked as if PTSD occurred in 15 to 20 percent (about one in five) of cancer survivors who had been through aggressive treatments, such as bone marrow transplants. However, further studies have indicated that most patients experience a milder version of posttraumatic stress, with some of the symptoms but not the full-blown picture of nightmares, anxiety, depression, flashbacks, and emotional "numbness." Dr. William Redd and his colleagues at Mount Sinai Medical Center found that about 15 percent of adult survivors of bone marrow transplants have full-blown PTSD, with some symptoms present in another 10 percent. A quarter of children who had been through difficult cancer treatments, as well as their mothers, showed posttraumatic signs a year later.

If you are experiencing any of these symptoms, you should seek help (see Chapter 6). Cognitive-behavioral therapy is effective in treating PTSD by reducing the response to the painful memories. Antianxiety medications may also be necessary.

Researchers are beginning to study persons with PTSD with brain scans. Using positron emission tomography (PET) and functional magnetic resonance imaging (fMRI), they are determining how traumatic memories are processed and in what areas of the brain. So far, the limbic system, which plays an important role in emotions, memory, learning, and behavior, appears to be involved. With Dr. Joy Hirsch, a neuroscientist at Memorial Sloan-Kettering Cancer Center, my group is studying Holocaust survivors who have developed cancer or have experienced a loss that seems to reactivate old, repressed, painful memories. It is likely that PTSD will turn out to be a window to understanding much more about the "hard-wiring" of the emotion of anxiety, effective and ineffective ways of coping with it, and who is more vulnerable to developing PTSD after a traumatic event.

SEX AND FERTILITY AFTER CANCER

Sexuality is a critical area of human life. From the early teenage years and onward, sexuality helps shape one's self-identity as a person capable of an intimate relationship with another human being and one who has the capacity to have a family and children. Both the psychological and physical aspects of sexuality may be impaired by cancer and its treatments. Both can have devastating effects on survivors, particularly on those who are young and just beginning to form intimate relationships (see Chapter 9).

I recall a young woman, Nina, who, in the course of a workup for infertility, was found to have uterine cancer, requiring a hysterectomy and the removal of her ovaries. The courage she and her husband displayed in confronting this painful reality was truly remarkable. They explored alternatives and were able to find a woman of the same ethnic group to serve as a surrogate mother (providing eggs) and to carry a pregnancy using the husband's sperm (the egg was fertilized in vitro). They now have a healthy little girl, who provides a happy ending to what originally appeared to be a painful, irretrievable loss.

Sometimes the loss is clearly physical: impotence following the cutting of pelvic nerves during prostatectomy (removal of the prostate); premature menopause and infertility in women after surgery or chemotherapy; infertility in teenage boys and men following treatment for leukemia, lymphoma, or testicular cancer. Today, as mentioned earlier, men and adolescent boys are given the opportunity to bank sperm prior to beginning high-dose chemotherapy for Hodgkin's disease, non-Hodgkin's lymphoma, acute leukemia, and testicular cancer. For a lot of men, this option reduces somewhat their sense of loss. Perhaps it is only a matter of time until similar banking of women's ova (eggs) can be done as well.

Even when the treatment has had no direct impact on the body's ability to function sexually, psychological effects can make it hard for survivors to see themselves as sexually attractive and desirable. It is not unusual for survivors to shun intimate relationships, particularly new ones. Common thoughts are: "What do I say when I undress and the scars show? How can I tell, yet how can I *not* tell, and be honest with someone I like a lot?" The inner loss of confidence in one's sexual identity can be as powerful a deterrent to returning to normal sexuality as an actual physical impairment of function.

The major issues for cancer survivors have been well described by Dr. Sarah Auchincloss, a psychiatrist. She points out that as a survivor you are simultaneously dealing with these psychological and physical aspects. The threat to life that cancer and its treatments present puts sex temporarily on a back burner. For six months to a year after finishing cancer treatment, the risk to your life is the framing experience. As Dr. Auchincloss says, "You can't pull your sex life out of the cancer frame too early." It is reassuring to recognize that the low or absent desire for sex in the early survival period is not unusual and represents the psyche's recovery from a trauma. It's like having been in a car crash and you come home feeling battered, bloodied, and shaken up, and your spouse or partner wants to have sex. You're ready to snap, "Are you out of your mind?"

How and when to get back to sex, even if it may not be as vigorous or satisfying as before the illness, is important. The pattern mentioned earlier is common. Couples are fearful: The healthy partner fears hurting the survivor, and the survivor interprets the lack of sexual advances from the partner as rejection.

These issues are rarely brought up by the doctors in follow-up visits. And they may not be brought up by the survivor, who views them as too trivial to "bother the doctor with." Wrong! They should be discussed, and if need be, the patient can be referred to a sex counselor or a support group composed of others who have been through a similar cancer experience.

One breast surgeon has an unequivocal "do ask" policy. At a follow-up visit, six months or so after mastectomy, he asks the patient about a return to sex; if the answer is an embarrassed no, he takes out his prescription pad and writes "Sex tonight." This breaks the ice with humor, but it also says to the patient and her partner that it is okay to have sex.

Auchincloss feels that women, as cancer survivors, feel less sexual for quite a while, though they may want to be held and feel closeness. She says:

> Women often push themselves to try to be sexual again faster than they want to be because they're worried about their husband or partner. It's similar to what often happens after pregnancy. A lot of women who are pregnant and nursing will happily tell you that they feel they wouldn't mind not having sex for a long time, because their testosterone level is practically zero after nursing for six months. But they have sex sooner because they feel it keeps the relationship from falling apart.

But what may be even more important to the male partner than sex, according to Auchincloss, is having back in his life "a woman who is not anxious all the time and who accepts her own body as it is, rather than a woman who is constantly turning to him to cheer her up about it."

When the problem has a direct physiological basis, sex counselors who are experienced at working with people with cancer and cancer survivors, as well as medical specialists such as gynecologists and urologists, can help you find a solution to a sexual or fertility problem. Dr. Leslie Schover, a psychologist, has written booklets for men and women on sexual issues, available from the American Cancer Society's national or local offices. (See Resources.) Depending on the specific problem, hormones, vaginal creams, a surgical procedure, or a sexual therapy technique might be recommended (see Chapter 9).

One valuable resource, not widely known, is an organization started by Dr. Lucy Waletzky, a psychiatrist and a major advocate for attention to the human side of cancer. Dr. Waletzky recognized several years ago that people with disabilities had few chances for normal dating and finding partners. She founded DATE-ABLE to create opportunities for those who might otherwise find it difficult to seek and find others with whom they might share an intimate relationship. DATE-ABLE has spread from Washington, D.C., to other cities and serves those with disabilities as an important source for maintaining self-esteem and sexual self-identity. While DATE-ABLE is open to people with any long-term disability, it is of particular interest to cancer survivors with disabilities from their surgical treatments who might otherwise be socially isolated.

RESOURCES FOR SURVIVORS

Increasing numbers of resources have been developed that offer assistance in all the main areas of life: physical, psychological, social, work, and sexual. The National Cancer Institute (1-800-4-CANCER) and the American Cancer Society (1-800-ACS-2345) are good first calls for advice. The Post-Treatment Resource Program at Memorial Sloan-Kettering Cancer Center in New York, directed by social worker Karrie Zampini, serves as a center for information and advice in all these areas. Cancer Care, Inc., also in New York, under Diane Blum's direction, is increasingly using telephone and telecommunication to provide advice and guidance on issues of concern to survivors. Y-Me is a national organization with a hot line for giving advice. SHARE in New York and Gilda's Clubs in many cities are excellent organizations that can help you find resources in your own community (see Resources).

The National Coalition for Cancer Survivorship is a growing, powerful voice for advocacy, based in Washington, D.C. Membership provides access to its newsletter, publications, and telephone contact persons. Its publications are outstanding on specific issues, such as work discrimination.

National advocacy groups for survivors of breast and ovarian cancer and, more recently, prostate and lung cancer suggest that people are recognizing the value of the grassroots, personal support given by other people with the same problems. These groups provide hope, personal meaning, a sense of control, and the all-important social support, which not only will enrich the quality of your life but may improve your physical health as well.

STAYING HEALTHY

I've changed my whole diet since I was ill. No more bacon cheeseburgers and fries! I eat a lot less fat, a lot more fiber, and plenty of fruits and vegetables. Not only have I lost some weight but, more important, I'm trying my best to keep from getting a recurrence of my cancer.

—Irma, who was treated successfully
for colon cancer

Since I finished my treatment, I've been tired all the time. A nurse at the hospital suggested I embark on a walking program. So I started small, and I've been building up little by little each week. Now, I'm starting to have more energy, and I'm not as short of breath as I used to be.

—Bernie, a lung cancer survivor

My doctor told me I'm cancer free. I feel like I could live another twenty to thirty years, so I'd better start taking care of myself. I've always been a real sun worshiper. I could lie out in the sun for hours. Now, I keep covered when the sun is out and I put on sunblock.

—Dawn, a melanoma survivor.

Jim is a busy storeowner and father of two teenage boys. At forty-five, he developed a scratchy throat and hoarseness that didn't go away. He tried the usual cough syrups and believed he had sinus trouble. However, when a doctor looked at his larynx, it showed an early cancer on the vocal cord. He underwent radiation and, fortunately, did not lose his voice box.

After the treatment was finished, the whole family breathed easier, though not without lingering concern for his continuing good health. Jim, who had smoked cigarettes since his twenties, cut down on his smoking when he learned the diagnosis, using nicotine gum. But he became concerned about his sons and their friends, who were at an age when the "Marlboro Country" is most enticing. He spoke with them honestly and allowed his feelings and paternal caring to help make the case that it is far easier never to start smoking than to endure a cancer illness and suffer through withdrawal. Jim also persuaded his wife that they had to be role models; children whose parents smoke are most likely to take up this habit. The experience with cancer of the larynx served as a wake-up call to correct health habits for all the members of this family.

After successfully running the gauntlet of treatments for a particular cancer, cancer survivors want to pursue health habits and practices that will keep them well. This dimension of the human side—how we can affect our risk of cancer and its course—encompasses health habits such as avoiding or quitting smoking, maintaining a good diet, moderating alcohol consumption, engaging in regular exercise, limiting sexual contacts, and avoiding exposure to the sun's harmful ultraviolet rays.

CANCER SCREENING TESTS

Staying healthy includes observing screening recommendations, such as the American Cancer Society guidelines regarding the Papanicolaou (Pap) test for cervical cancer, mammography for breast cancer, and the prostate specific antigen (PSA) blood test for prostate cancer. These screening tests are just as important after one has had cancer as before.

In April 1999, the National Cancer Institute reported that the rates of new cancer cases and deaths for all cancers combined, as well as for most of the top ten cancer sites, declined between 1990 and 1996 in the United States. The report was truly good news, indicating that we are beginning to win the war on cancer. The only caveat was that adolescent smoking is increasing, which foretells a concern about whether lung cancer will continue to decline.

The dramatic decline in cervical cancer in the Western world is attributed to the wide use of Pap tests in women's routine gynecological care. Moreover, the National Cancer Institute reported the first drop in mortality from breast cancer, beginning in 1991, attributed to the increased use of mammograms by women in the United States. This practice has led to an earlier diagnosis and, therefore, treatment of more curable tumors with a good prognosis. Another important screening test is the PSA test for prostate cancer in men. It is usually recommended beginning at age fifty, but it may be given at a younger age for men with a family history of prostate cancer.

Beginning at age fifty, both men and women need to have regular colonoscopy, a procedure that checks the colon for precancerous growths called polyps. Your doctor should determine how frequently you need colonoscopy based on your personal or genetic risk for colon cancer.

LIFESTYLE AND SURVIVING CANCER

The long-term lifestyle issues that are important for cancer survivors are outlined below. These guidelines are important, not only for your own health, but also for the health of your family members. As a survivor, you have a powerful bully pulpit from which to urge your family members to change behaviors that are placing them at greater risk for cancer. Not only can you speak out as an advocate for cancer prevention, but your family is probably more receptive to listening now that one member of the family has been treated for cancer. The cancer diagnosis and treatment of one family member create a significant opportunity, which can be grasped by the entire family, to initiate healthier lifestyle changes to prevent cancer.

TOBACCO USE AND CIGARETTE SMOKING

Cigarette smoking is the single most preventable cause of premature death and disability in the United States, implicated in one of every six deaths. The statistics are telling: Cigarette smoking is related to 21 percent of all deaths from coronary artery disease; 30 percent of cancer mortality (death rate); 87 percent of all lung cancer deaths; and 82 percent of deaths from emphysema and chronic pulmonary disease.

These facts reflect smoking-related deaths in our country today, despite the fact that the association of cigarette smoking with lung cancer was announced by the Surgeon General of the United States in 1964 and that the relation between smoking and coronary artery disease and chronic lung disease has been clear for a long time. It is distressing to note that between 1965 and 1991, rather than dropping, the number of smoking-related deaths actually rose for cancer of the lung, mouth and throat, larynx (voice box), and esophagus. Smokers also bear a greater risk of cancer of the bladder and, possibly, of the kidney and pancreas.

For many years, it was difficult to get people to listen to warnings of the dangers of smoking. Often, nonsmokers were ostracized or ridiculed when they complained about breathing in a smoky room or tried to exhort others not to smoke. But recently, a turnaround has occurred in the United States: The social stigma today is *against* smoking and smokers. Laws banning smoking in public places have been put in place, and they are actually enforced. Smokers today must smoke in isolation or bear considerable criticism from nonsmokers. Nevertheless, the risk of cancer from smoking is rising in women and minority populations. Dr. Ellen Gritz, an outstanding researcher of smoking-related cancers at M.D. Anderson Cancer Center in Texas, has sent the important message that people who stop smoking before age fifty reduce their risk of death from *all* causes (including cancer) by 50 percent; if they do not resume smoking, by age sixty-four, their mortality is similar to that of people who never smoked. In fact, even individuals who have *had* cancer and quit smoking benefit in terms of better outcome of their cancer and longer survival.

The social cost in health care is so enormous that several state governments have initiated lawsuits that have been successful in obtaining settlements from the major tobacco companies to reimburse the states for the health care burden on society caused by smoking; they have also been able to curtail cigarette advertising geared toward young people. The addictive quality of cigarettes, long recognized but denied by manufacturers, has finally been acknowledged. Chewing tobacco has a high potential to cause cancer in the mouth. Often teenage boys start chewing tobacco to emulate professional athletes in baseball whom they see "chewing and spitting," not realizing that most are chewing gum! Cigar smoking raises the risk of lip and mouth cancer. While less worrisome than cigarettes, cigars, too, should be avoided, despite their recent cachet with celebrities featured on the covers of magazines for cigar smokers.

Some of the most exciting psychological research in oncology has gone into promoting ways to help smokers stop and to help teenagers resist smoking in the first place. Those who start to smoke after the teen years rarely become severely habituated smokers. The good news is that the percentage of adults who smoke has diminished (between 1965 and 1993) from 42 percent to 25 percent. However, there has been a plateau in the drop-off. Billboard ads appealing to adolescents and ads aimed at women have contributed to the increased smoking in these groups. Doctors, who are important gatekeepers for monitoring patients' lifestyles and habits, were slow to ask patients routinely about smoking, and it has taken a major campaign to encourage primary-care physicians and specialists to ask their patients whether they smoke and to offer assistance in stopping.

Some people simply stop cold and do not smoke again, but because the nicotine in cigarettes is addictive, it is a difficult habit for many people to break in this way. The treatments that work best combine nicotine replacement with support from a clinician and specific techniques to assist in stopping (for example, scheduled smoking with longer and longer intervals between cigarettes). Nicotine gum and patches can help you stop smoking by gradually reducing your intake of nicotine and, therefore, your addiction to it. Recognizing the frequent relationship between depression and addiction

Figure 2. Cancer Mortality for Women★

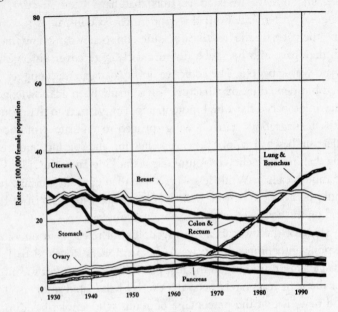

*Per 100,000, age-adjusted to the 1970 U.S. standard population.
†Uterus cancer death rates are for uterine cervix and uterine corpus combined.
Note: Due to changes in ICD coding, numerator information has changed over time. Rates for cancer of the uterus, ovary, lung and bronchus, and colon and rectum are affected by these coding changes.
American Cancer Society, Surveillance Research, 1999. Data source: *Vital Statistics of the United States,* 1998.
© 1999, American Cancer Society, Inc.

to tobacco, the antidepressant bupropion (Zyban) is often added to stop-smoking routines. It appears that chronically depressed individuals are actually smoking as a way of seeking relief from their depression. For this group of smokers, it is hard, if not impossible, to stop smoking without the addition of an antidepressant.

Dr. Jamie Ostroff, chief, Behavioral Sciences Service, in our research group, has used the diagnosis of cancer as a time to approach not only the newly diagnosed patient at our hospital, but also family members who smoke. She views the time when people are confronting illness as a "teachable moment," because they are more willing to listen to information about changing a behavior that exposes all family members to risk. New research is also exploring the connection between genetic vulnerability and exposure to tobacco. It

Figure 3 Cancer Mortality for Men*.

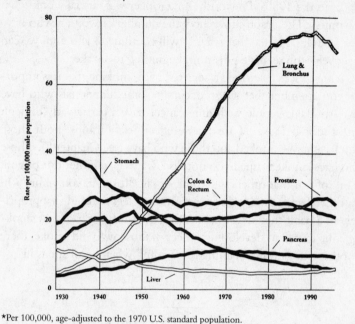

*Per 100,000, age-adjusted to the 1970 U.S. standard population.
Note: Due to changes in ICD coding, numerator information has changed over time. Rates for cancer of the liver, lung and bronchus, and colon and rectum are affected by these coding changes.
American Cancer Society, Surveillance Research, 1999. Data source: *Vital Statistics of the United States*, 1998.
© 1999, American Cancer Society, Inc.

may be that some people can smoke with less cancer risk because of their genetic makeup, while others, because of their genetic makeup, increase their cancer risk by smoking. We hope that studying these differences will one day lead us to a better understanding of what causes some people but not others to develop tobacco-related cancers.

The survival advantage of stopping smoking is especially great for those with lung cancer, in whom stopping reduces the chance of a new tumor developing. Many women do not recognize the fact that the mortality from cancer for women is now higher for lung cancer than for breast cancer (see Figure 2). The epidemic of lung cancer surfaced in men in the 1930s, about twenty to forty years after cigarette smoking became popular among men in the United States (see Figure 3). Large numbers of women began to smoke in the 1920s, and the deaths from lung cancer among women began to appear in the 1950s. Previously, lung cancer was virtually unknown in women. The graph shows how the number of women who have died from lung cancer has risen; it will continue to rise until we can effectively stop teenage girls from beginning to smoke.

Lung cancer is so often associated with smoking that it is important to remember that it also occurs in some individuals who have never smoked. People with lung cancer have a particularly difficult time today because of this cause-effect relationship—both those who have never smoked and those who have (see Chapter 8). Those who have smoked usually do not discuss this fact, either out of guilt or out of fear that others will think or say, "It serves you right." On the other hand, those who never smoked feel accused inappropriately of a habit they never had. Although it may be true that smoking contributed to developing cancer in those who did smoke, there is nothing to gain in "blaming the victim" when he or she is ill.

ALCOHOL AND CANCER

People often do not realize that excessive alcohol intake (above about 4 oz per day) exposes the tissues of the mouth, throat, larynx, esophagus, and liver to substances that increase the risk of cancer in these sites. Public education has been minimal about these risks, perhaps because alcohol is so much a part of our culture and because it is hard to define what constitutes an excessive intake. Also, little information has been given to the public about the increased risk of cancer that results from combined cigarette smoking and excessive alcohol consumption. It is not known exactly what the interaction between the two is, but the risk of cancer shoots up exponentially in heavy users of both alcohol and tobacco. It is common for heavy drinkers to be heavy smokers as well. These individuals are often people who have significant psychological problems, which lead them to excessive intake of cigarettes and alcohol. Family problems result from the alcohol addiction.

Unfortunately, individuals who have severe alcohol and smoking problems are often resistant to interventions. Families need help in getting these members to counseling and to Alcoholics Anonymous or Nicotine Anonymous. The risks are high and the health hazard clear if both habits continue unabated. A major percentage of tumors in the head and neck region occur in people who have a history of heavy alcohol and tobacco use. These individuals also are likely to have poor nutrition and vitamin deficiencies, which further add to cancer risk. The exact mechanism by which alcohol changes cells to make them vulnerable to cancer isn't known, but it may interfere with the ability of genes to repair the DNA of healthy cells, impair the metabolism of vitamin A, or suppress the immune system. For those who have had a tumor of the head or neck region, it is an advantage to stop smoking and reduce alcohol intake to lower the risk of developing a new tumor or increasing the risk of the original cancer coming back.

DIET AND OBESITY

According to the American Cancer Society, about one-third of cancer deaths that occur in the United States each year are due to dietary factors. The dietary guidelines for avoidance of cancer, as well as heart disease, are quite clear. A low-fat diet is common to both. A diet rich in fiber can help protect against colon cancer, as can a moderate-to-light intake of animal protein, with plenty of vegetables and fruits. (Although the genetic risk of colon cancer is important, diet and physical activity may help to modify that risk.) In 1992 the U.S. Department of Agriculture developed the Food Guide Pyramid, which shows foods divided into six groups and recommends the number of servings of foods from each group per day. The fats and sweets at the top of the pyramid should be eaten most sparingly. (The recommended servings for each food category are given in Figure 4.)

The American Cancer Society revised its nutrition guidelines in 1996 (see Table 5); the new guidelines are consistent with the U.S. Department of Agriculture Food Guide Pyramid. Most foods should be chosen from plant sources, such as fruits and vegetables, whole grains, and legumes. From scientific studies, we know that consumption of green and dark yellow vegetables, cruciferous vegetables (those in the cabbage family, such as broccoli, cauliflower, cabbage, and Brussels sprouts), soy products, and beans protects from cancer of the gastrointestinal and respiratory systems. Grains, which are high in fiber content, provide many minerals and reduce the risk of colon cancer. It appears prudent to maintain a high-fiber intake. High-fat foods, especially those derived from animal meats, increase the risk of colon, endometrial, and prostate cancer. Whether fats increase breast cancer risk is less clear at this point, but while the jury is out, it's probably best to limit your intake of animal protein and fat. Some research suggests that foods or supplements containing antioxidants, such as vitamins A, C, and E and the minerals zinc and selenium, may help prevent cancer. Antioxidants prevent the production of *free radicals,* which are chemical substances that may promote abnormal cell growth.

Figure 4. The Food Guide Pyramid

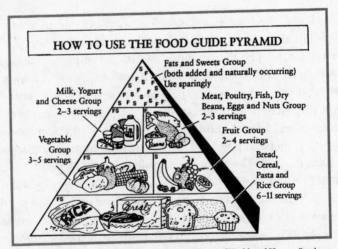

Source: U.S. Department of Agriculture/U.S. Department of Health and Human Services

TABLE 5

AMERICAN CANCER SOCIETY
NUTRITION GUIDELINES (1996)

CHOOSE MOST OF THE FOODS YOU EAT
FROM PLANT SOURCES.

LIMIT YOUR INTAKE OF HIGH FAT FOODS,
PARTICULARLY FROM ANIMAL SOURCES.

BE PHYSICALLY ACTIVE: ACHIEVE AND
MAINTAIN A HEALTHY WEIGHT.

LIMIT YOUR CONSUMPTION OF ALCOHOLIC
BEVERAGES, IF YOU DRINK AT ALL.

American Cancer Society Facts and Figures, 1997

WEIGHT CONTROL

Obesity, often linked to insufficient exercise as well as diet, increases the risk of colon, rectal, prostate, kidney, and endometrial cancer, as well as of breast cancer in postmenopausal women. While less is known as to whether nutrition and exercise promote longer survival after a cancer illness, it is likely that they act in similar fashion as in cancer risk. For patients with cancer, especially survivors who want to stay healthy and prevent recurrence, maintaining normal weight and exercising are recommended. This advice is important for women who have had breast cancer, who often gain weight during chemotherapy and have trouble returning to their normal weight. Weight control, through diet and exercise, has salutary effects, both physically and psychologically.

EXERCISE

Exercise itself may be protective against cancer in ways we don't yet understand. Some studies have suggested that people who exercise more have a lower risk of colon cancer. We do know that exercise helps to decrease depression and anxiety. In a study of women following surgery for breast cancer, one-third of the women who exercised found that their anxiety and depression were reduced.

"Walking is one of the most appropriate aerobic activities for adults with breathing problems, depression, anxiety, and fatigue," according to Donna J. Wilson, clinical nurse specialist at Memorial Sloan-Kettering Cancer Center. It is simple and straightforward, requiring no special skill, setting, or equipment other than a good pair of shoes. Walking is also one of the exercises least likely to cause or aggravate musculoskeletal problems. "The catch," Wilson says, "is you have to get out there and do it constantly." (See Table 6 for Wilson's walking program.)

TABLE 6

SIX-WEEK WALKING PROGRAM

Developed by Donna J. Wilson, Clinical Nurse Specialist,
Memorial Sloan-Kettering Cancer Center

THIS IS A SELF-PACED AND INDIVIDUALIZED
PROGRAM TO MEET YOUR NEEDS AND FITNESS LEVEL.

WEEK	DURATION	FREQUENCY
1	5 MINUTES	3–5 TIMES/WEEK
2	10 MINUTES	3–5 TIMES/WEEK
3	15 MINUTES	3–5 TIMES/WEEK
4	20 MINUTES	3–5 TIMES/WEEK
5	25 MINUTES	3–5 TIMES/WEEK
6	30 MINUTES	3–5 TIMES/WEEK

BEFORE YOU BEGIN
Wear comfortable clothing and
sneakers or walking shoes.

WARM-UP

Take 5 deep breaths; as you breathe in, stretch your arms
over your head, and as you breathe out, lower your arms.

◆

Start at a comfortable pace and gradually
increase your pace after 2 minutes.

DURING YOUR WALK

Use your arms for balance, gently swinging them.

◆

As you walk, focus on exhaling,
breathing out through pursed lips;
breathing in will come naturally.

◆

Monitor your exercise intensity (use a scale from 1 to 10)
1–2: no stress, very comfortable
4–6: you notice the increased effort, but you're not tired
8–10: you're exhausted; STOP and sit down
Try to maintain your exercise intensity
level in the 4–6 range.

COOL DOWN

Spend the last 1 to 2 minutes of your walk
gradually slowing down.

STRETCH

Stretch after your walk when your muscles are warm and
pliable. Hold stretches for 10 to 15 seconds and breathe naturally. Be sure to stretch your calves and lower back gently.

MAKE A COMMITMENT

When you wake up every day, think about
when you will walk.

GET IN THE HABIT

Do not worry about speed, just focus on
walking as an everyday event.

◆

Seeing your progress will make you—and keep you—
enthusiastic about your program. Walking is the easiest
route to better health, more energy,
and a refreshed state of mind.

SUN EXPOSURE

Sunlight is critical to health, yet too much exposure to sunlight is linked to skin cancer and malignant melanoma. However, some people are more susceptible than others: those with fair skin and blue eyes, who freckle easily, and who have a tendency to sunburn rather than tan. Australia, because of its sunny climate and fair-skinned people, has led the way to reducing the frequency of melanoma by launching campaigns to reduce sun tanning and sun exposure. A similar campaign is under way in the United States. But the most addicted "sun worshipers" have a strong psychological need for sun tanning. It is important for them to see the big picture: that it is more important to stay healthy than to exhibit the false glow of health a suntan offers. The Melanoma Update, produced for patients and their families at Memorial Sloan-Kettering, outlines rules for being sun-smart (see Table 7).

Many of us have normal spots on the skin that are benign, such as moles and freckles. Sometimes these normal spots undergo a malignant change to melanoma. Simple rules called the ABCD's of melanoma can help you identify a suspicious spot (see Table 8). Anyone with lots of freckles and moles might do well to be examined on a regular basis by a dermatologist, who can detect changes more easily. Some dermatologists take full-body pictures to record the appearance of the moles and freckles. A suspected change can be compared with an earlier picture.

TABLE 7. AVOIDING SKIN CANCER

1. RULES FOR SUMMER SUN

Choose sun-protective clothing.

Apply sunscreen.

Avoid sunburn.

Never work on a tan.

Avoid prolonged exposure to intense sunlight.

Cover up with a hat and shirt.

Never lie out in the sun.

Seek shade while engaging in outdoor activities.

2. USE OF SUNSCREEN

Apply sunscreen to all parts of the body not protected by clothing.

Use a sunscreen with a Sun Protection Factor (SPF) of 15 or higher; higher is better.

Judge sunscreen efficacy by SPF, not by price.

In choosing a sunscreen, ultraviolet light (UVA) protection is a bonus.

For longer exposures, choose a water-resistant or "sports" formulation.

Apply sunscreen before going outdoors.

Reapply sunscreen after swimming or working up a sweat.

TABLE 8

THE ABCD'S OF MELANOMA

A. Asymmetry is characteristic of a melanoma, whereas a mole is usually round.

B. Borders are usually uneven on a melanoma, whereas a mole has smooth, even borders.

C. Color in a mole tends to differ from that in a melanoma: Moles are a uniform brown color, whereas a mole that is turning into a melanoma is becoming a different shade of brown.

D. Diameter is important. Common moles are small, while melanomas tend to be larger than the size of a pencil eraser. People who have many moles or freckles should examine themselves regularly and have someone else examine their backs. Dermatologists are now routinely taking photos of individuals with many freckles and moles, so that any suspicious skin changes will be seen by comparing these pictures over time.

SEXUAL CONTACTS

Women's magazines and other media are now publicizing the fact that a virus, the human papillomavirus (HPV), which is transmitted through sexual contact, is the major cause of cervical cancer. Routine Pap smears can pick up early abnormal precancerous cervical changes, and early treatment prevents cervical cancer from developing. Even if cervical cancer develops, when treated early it is curable. A tragedy in developing countries is that women who don't have access to Pap tests come in for medical care at a late stage of the disease, when the cervical cancer has advanced to an incurable stage. Careful monitoring for cervical changes is the best advice, plus the use of condoms to reduce exposure.

THE BOTTOM LINE

What does all this mean? Put together, research suggests that behaviors are important in avoiding cancer and in surviving it. Lifestyle, particularly diet and exercise, as well as habits, which include tobacco use, excessive alcohol intake, excessive sun exposure, and sexual contacts that expose one to sexually transmitted diseases, put people at greater risk of specific cancers. These preventive measures are personal decisions, and they appear to be of greater importance than the worries about elevated levels of radon or exposure to toxins in the environment. Unfortunately, environmental carcinogens capture the public's attention, at the expense of recognizing that our "personal" environment—our habits and exposures—may be more important.

We now know much more about preventing cancer than we ever did in the past. It is unfortunate that the knowledge we have doesn't translate easily into changing habits that put us at risk. If prevention were a pill to take, people would comply far better than when they have to give up a favorite habit. It is often difficult to change a habit that is part of our lifestyle. A great deal of help is available through smoking cessation, weight loss, and Twelve-Step programs, as well as nutritional counseling, to facilitate life changes that can profoundly affect health and survival.

In addition, attention ought to be paid to the American Cancer Society's guidelines for screening for certain types of cancer: mammography for breast cancer, Pap smears for cervical cancer, fecal blood examination and colonoscopy for colorectal cancer, and the PSA test for prostate cancer. These measures can lead to early diagnosis should a tumor be present without symptoms (see Table 9). Although it isn't desirable to become preoccupied with fears of cancer, common sense in lifestyle and health practices should prevail, with the hope that recurrence of a treated cancer or development of a new cancer can be prevented.

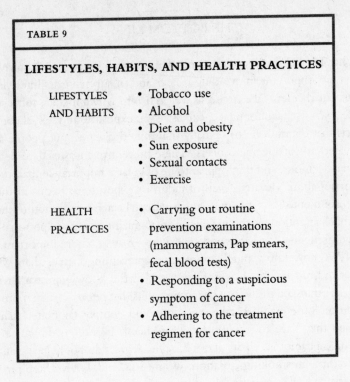

TABLE 9

LIFESTYLES, HABITS, AND HEALTH PRACTICES

LIFESTYLES AND HABITS	• Tobacco use • Alcohol • Diet and obesity • Sun exposure • Sexual contacts • Exercise
HEALTH PRACTICES	• Carrying out routine prevention examinations (mammograms, Pap smears, fecal blood tests) • Responding to a suspicious symptom of cancer • Adhering to the treatment regimen for cancer

13

THE GOAL IS CONTROL

*Each second we live is a new and unique moment of
the universe, a moment that never was before and never
will be again.*

—Pablo Casals

*My reactions, since my lung cancer came back, are like
a roller-coaster ride. One day, I go shopping like crazy
and buy new clothes and plan a thousand things to do.
The next day, panic sets in, and I start cleaning out my
closets and giving everything away.*

—Georgia, a fifty-seven-year-old
florist with lung cancer

*You know how I would trip out every time I had to
have scans after my breast cancer treatment last year? It
was like I lived in fear the other shoe would drop. Well,
it has. The cancer's back and this time it's in my liver.
The hardest thing for me right now is not knowing
what's coming next. I'm going to start a new treatment
without knowing whether it will work. My hope is that
it will control the cancer until something really good
comes along; new things become available all the time.
It's so weird. I know the cancer's back, and I have to
work with the doctors to control it. But the really
depressing thing is I know I won't go back to my old
self again. I have to live with it.*

—Trish, a young woman who just got
news of spread of her cancer

*I never thought I could take it if the cancer came back,
but here I am, feeling good that the treatment has
shrunk the tumors in my lungs. I think the way I manage is that I just ratchet down the meaning of what's
happening until it is tolerable.*

—Paul, a thirty-eight-year-old architect whose
colon cancer recurred in his lungs

These quotations express the dismay, fear, and sadness that are
caused by the recurrence or spread of cancer, together with the
great uncertainty of the outcome of renewed treatments for a new
stage of disease. To hear that "the cancer has come back" is devastating news. It means facing treatments again after assuming all was
well and hoping it would never come back. It means wondering,
"Will the new treatment work?" and, if it does, "How long will it
work?" It means saying to yourself, "Maybe this cancer can still be
controlled with the treatments available until something *really* good
comes along that will zap it and get me back to where I was." The
feelings of fear, regret, and uncertainty, tinged with hope for a new
treatment, are all mixed together, and the one that dominates varies
on the basis of the current news and how you're feeling physically.

People who learn that their cancer has come back go through
similar emotional reactions to those they went through when they
learned of the first cancer diagnosis: shock ("It can't be true"), turmoil ("I can't face this"), and finally adaptation ("The doctor tells
me that there are treatments for this stage, and I better get on with
them"). The difference, however, is that the turmoil and adaptation
phases are now often tinged with more sadness. The anxiety that
new treatments must be faced again and, especially, the dread that
their outcome is uncertain add to the new emotional burdens. The
thought of resuming treatments after a period of good health is overwhelming at first.

But the reality is, and it is important to keep this in mind if you
are faced with this situation, that there *are* effective treatments for
recurrent disease. In fact, it is for disease at this level that new treatments are being discovered and tried every day. There is every rea-

son to hope that a new drug or treatment "in the pipeline" will emerge to truly turn cancer around at this stage. This is particularly true right now with breast and prostate tumors, for which hormonal and immune therapies are being developed. New chemotherapy for other tumors, like colon and lung cancers, is also becoming available.

The good news about the bad news is that, indeed, in recent years, cancer has become a chronic disease for many people. Doctors treat many patients with cancer not for cure, but for control. The old "alive or dead" equation that went with cancer no longer applies. When cancer has recurred after a period of health, or progressed to the point that control is the goal, the issues are those of coping with a chronic illness that continues to pose a threat to life. Natalie Spingarn, mentioned earlier in this book as a twenty-four-year survivor of metastatic breast cancer, put it well when she said that she embodied a new category of survivor, one who was living "a different kind of life." She meant that she made concessions to some aspects of chronic illness by cutting back on certain activities, but she increased others that dealt with advocacy for patients with cancer.

One difficult aspect of dealing with a recurrence of cancer was expressed by Trish, quoted at the beginning of this chapter: "I know I won't go back to my old self again. I have to live with it." It is unhappy news at any age, but it is more distressing to young people, whose life awaits them. They are surprised by their anger and envy of healthy peers even though it is understandable. Expressions like these are common: "I can't help being envious of people I see who are exercising and going about their normal lives." "I don't ask 'why me?' because there's no good answer, but it's just so hard." Living with a chronic illness is colored with sadness about lost good health and the reality that this is likely the way life is going to be for some time.

Many more people live with chronic illness today than ever before in our history. Living with chronic illness may make you feel like an alien in a foreign land. In his book *In the Country of Illness,* Robert Lipsyte gives a remarkably honest and entertaining account of his journey to Malady, the country of illness. His writing is filled with "tumor humor" (a critical piece of baggage to carry along on the journey, he says). His encounters with the natives (the doctors and nurses) of Malady and their strange language (med speak) and customs (health care today) are described with wisdom and advice for the traveler to Malady, particularly for the second journey and a stay "in-country." Lipsyte had surgery and chemotherapy for testicular cancer and then developed cancer in his other testicle, which took him for a long visit to Malady.

In addition to the emotions and issues described earlier, Lipsyte brings attention to the unmentionable, anger-tinged issue of *money* in Malady. The cost of care today is enormous, and the role of health insurance is crucial for getting cancer treatment or sometimes *not* getting it. He points out that people may reveal their scars at dinner parties but they never talk about how much their operation cost. However, people do commiserate more openly today about medical costs and health plans. Lipsyte abhors the fact that with illness, money too often secures greater comfort and care, dignity, and even survival. Bills from hospitals come with not-so-gentle reminders, at a time when just keeping the insurance forms filled out is a full-time job. One woman who had lengthy and ongoing treatment for breast cancer said, "I just gave up. The bills came and I put them all in a basket, unopened. I simply didn't feel that I could deal with them."

Today, some people make a career out of taking medical bills, sending in the claims forms, and fighting with the insurance companies to get the reimbursement. The latter is another emotional burden of our current system. Why should you have to fight to get reimbursed when you paid the insurance premiums faithfully, both long before and during the illness?

Lipsyte suggests, "We need a Patients' Union, something between the serious and useful approach of the Consumers Union and the muscular intimidation of the Teamsters' Union in their Jimmy Hoffa heyday, that will rate doctors and medical facilities, provide a decent price structure and throw up a line of beefy picketers if we're gouged or treated badly. . . . Maybe it's time for a bedpan revolution, or at least an organization really dedicated to the needs of the sick and to those who love and take care of them."

For those who have a chronic illness, and therefore, a permanent home (an "in-country stay") in Malady, Lipsyte's words are cogent and honest: "Chronic diseases that require long-term medical care may also require long-term readjustments. Your relationships with your body, your environment, your family and friends may undergo enormous changes. Anxiety, fear and depression are common, often *indirect* results of the disease itself, but *direct* results of the rearrangements." Lipsyte underscores the importance of recognizing that distress is common, whether it results from illness or from the strains of "rearrangement," and that maintaining relationships to key people is a critical part of coping.

When cancer becomes a chronic illness, it may mean having to partially or fully give up work. Home becomes the locus of care and coping. It can be a dreary place if you live alone, or if you are left alone each day when everyone else in the household is working or at school. Money rears its ugly head here, too, because paying for help at home in the form of home health aides is expensive. The patients' union that Lipsyte suggested (a great idea) should protest loudly the inadequate attention that has been given by the government to the costs of care at home, especially now that hospital stays are so brief. Medicare and Medicaid do not provide sufficient help for homebound patients. More of these issues are discussed in Chapter 15, which deals with the stress on the family as its members become the primary caregivers.

The kinds of support that could be available in the community to help with coping are often lacking when patients are homebound, creating major problems. Many approaches are being explored now to see which methods lend themselves to helping people at home. At Memorial Sloan-Kettering, my colleagues and I are beginning a telephone support program for women with lung cancer who are homebound. We will compare a series of weekly telephone counseling sessions by a psychologist with a similar series using a video phone, in which the patient can hear—and see—the counselor, and the counselor can see the patient, allowing a better assessment of appearance for problems such as pain or depression. Another program, from Cabrini Hospital in New York, includes art therapy visits in the home, so that patients can express their feelings through art (see Chapter 9).

An innovative program was recently tested by Bruce Rybarczyk, a psychologist at Rush University in Chicago. Older adults with chronic illness received videotapes giving advice on nutrition, diet, exercise, and management of anxiety and depression using meditation and relaxation. Someone on the mental health team at the hospital phoned to follow up and check on patients' progress. Patients had fewer medical symptoms, slept better, and had a decrease in anxiety and depression as compared with a control group. They felt better, even though they didn't change their health habits very much. Patients also sought out additional information about practical self-help techniques, which likely gave them a sense of greater control over their situation. Rybarczyk speculated that the patients were able to look at their illness in a more constructive way.

Antonio, a seventy-year-old, retired cabinetmaker, found retirement with his wife a joy because he could putter around with his woodworking. In his leisure time, he made some lovely pieces of furniture for their home. At his annual physical checkup, his doctor found that he had signs of prostate cancer, confirmed by biopsy. Because the tumor was somewhat large, the doctors gave him hormonal therapy first, to decrease production of testosterone and shrink the tumor. Then they operated and removed his prostate. He did well, his energy returned, and all his checkups showed his prostate-specific antigen (PSA) level to be near zero. All his body scans were negative for signs of tumor spread. The life of retirement with winters in Florida returned to normal. Antonio felt secure except for the week before the six-month follow-up visits, when he could not sleep well and "felt nervous until the reports all came back."

At the three-year follow-up visit, the report came back with bad news. Antonio's PSA level had risen to 15, and his bone marrow scans showed two "hot spots" in the thigh and pelvic bones. While walking, he had noted some pain in his left hip. His doctor told him that the tumor had spread and that he needed to be placed back on hormonal treatment with Lupron and Casodex. This regimen caused the tumor to regress, and his PSA level fell. He developed troublesome hot flashes from the hormone therapy, side effects that were helped by the antidepressant drug sertraline (Zoloft). He received radiation therapy to his left hip and upper leg, which relieved the pain. His doctor assured him that new therapies were under development and that a chemotherapy regimen of Taxol and Estramustine was proving effective when tumors like his became unresponsive to the hormones, as eventually they did.

While Antonio and his wife had to adjust to his being under treatment all the time, they found that they could still pursue family activities with children and grandchildren and continued to winter in Florida. They felt optimistic that recurrent prostate cancer was receiving more scientific attention, which might lead to the discovery of new treatments in time. Antonio at seventy-three felt he could live out his life with this chronic disease.

Greta, a sixty-five-year-old mother of three grown children, a daughter and two sons, received news that the breast cancer for which she had been treated six years earlier had recurred in her lung. This meant that the cancer had now spread and that a new treatment was required. She had taken Tamoxifen for five years without bothersome side effects. It came as a shock when her annual checkup revealed several spots in her chest X ray. In addition, her Ca 27–29, a marker protein for breast cancer, had risen to 55, suggesting that the lung spots were metastases. She consulted a medical oncologist, who told her that there is a wide range of hormonal and chemotherapy drugs that work for metastatic breast cancer. She began on Arimidex, a hormone antagonist designed to deprive the cells of estrogen produced in the body's fat cells. Although she had no toxic side effects, the lung metastases did not shrink and the Ca 27–29 level continued to rise.

A shift was made to chemotherapy. Losing her hair and getting a wig took an emotional toll, but her primary complaint was the fatigue. Antinausea drugs given before the chemotherapy totally prevented her from getting sick from the treatments. The tumors got smaller after the second treatment, but after nine months there appeared to be a slight increase, and her Ca 27–29 level, which had fallen, again rose. Her doctor suggested that she participate in a Phase III clinical trial being conducted under the auspices of the National Cancer Institute. The study compared a standard treatment for this stage of cancer with a promising new high-dose chemotherapy regimen. The new treatment had been studied in Phase I, which meant that the dose, toxicity, and safety had been established, and Phase II trials showed that the drug was active against breast cancer. The Phase III trial was being offered to women in several centers to determine whether it was superior to the conventional treatment.

Greta agreed to participate in the trial, recognizing that, by random selection (made by the computer), she would receive either the present standard treatment or the new regimen, which might be better. She would get careful followup of her treatment and the care that goes with a carefully planned and conducted clinical trial. She was randomized to receive the standard treatment, and the tumor in her lung showed significant shrinkage. Her doctor assured her that if she needed further treatment, a range of third- and fourth-line treatments were available, as well as new agents currently under development. She found other longtime survivors of metastatic breast cancer in a support group she joined. They shared how their lives had changed, but they found ways to enjoy life in its altered form.

Gabriel was a busy fifty-three-year-old real estate salesman who was out every day in every kind of weather, doing his job. His dry cough seemed ordinary enough at the outset, but when it persisted he went to his doctor. It seemed impossible to him that he could have lung cancer, but that was what the doctor showed him on the X ray. Not only that, but the cancer had spread to his mediastinum (the space between the lungs) and to several vertebrae in his spine. He felt helpless and hopeless that anything could be done. He thought he should give up, "stop work and take a trip around the world. How do you live on borrowed time?" he asked. His initial response was tempered by his wife, who asserted, "Nonsense, you start your treatment immediately."

Gabriel's doctor showed him the shrinkage of the tumor in a chest X ray after three treatments with Taxol and cis-platin. He was encouraged to join a group of patients who also carried his diagnosis of Stage IV lung cancer. To his sur-prise, he found several in the group who had been receiving chemotherapy for over three years and were rearranging their lives. He also heard about their lively interest in new treatment trials and in the range of alternative therapies, about which they knew a lot. His spirits improved when he joined in their blend of humor one minute and serious talk the next. They sought a philosophical way to "hang in" and live with this chronic state, although it carried the constant threat of progression.

It is important to recognize also that some cancers grow so slowly that oncologists often elect not to treat them when they are discovered inadvertently and are causing no symptoms. Often years go by before symptoms develop that indicate the need to begin treatment. The common slow-growing cancers are low-grade prostate cancer, chronic lymphocytic leukemia, low-grade lym-phomas, and indolent metastatic breast cancer. These may be so slowly progressive that some older patients may never require treat-ment. This advice, on the surface, sounds reassuring; one might expect the person to say, "Thanks. I dodged that bullet and I'm con-tent to wait and see." However, perhaps the hardest thing to do, psy-chologically, is to do nothing at all. This course is very hard for some people, especially for those who want to be sure they have done everything that can be done. You are likely to be worried and upset about having cancer and letting it go untreated. You feel a lot of uncertainty, and your spirits are way down. It helps if your doctor can discuss why it is safer not to treat the condition: The side effects of treatment may make it a greater risk to life than withholding treatment.

There have also been major advances in the surgical treatment of metastatic tumors. Today, surgeons operate successfully to remove single metastatic tumors or occasionally several tumors in a single organ site. Colon cancers that recur with one or more tumors in the liver or lung may often be effectively removed, sometimes by laser surgery, which is minimally invasive, or by removing the lobe of the liver containing the tumor. Tumors in the lung are removed either by opening up the chest and taking out a part of the lobe that contains the tumor or by using the thoracoscope and taking out a wedge of the lobe that contains the tumor without opening the lung.

Single metastatic lesions in the brain are often removed. Radiation is then usually given to prevent growth of other tiny metastases that may be present. Bone metastases from breast cancer, which once were disabling and painful, can now be treated with a drug called pamidronate, which strengthens the bones and decreases pain, slows tumor growth, and reduces the possibility of fractures.

What can *you* do to make the human side of living with cancer at this stage easier? Acknowledge that this is a difficult period that will elicit mixed emotions varying from hopeful to hopeless, from confidence to insecurity, from fearful to feeling in control and on top of things, and from sadness to gratitude for being alive. How to cope is an individual matter, unique to each of us. It is a time when you fare best when you seek the best treatment, follow through with it, and get help for troubling physical symptoms. Remember that scientific progress, although often slow and difficult, is inevitable, and breakthroughs may occur in time for your benefit. Keeping these thoughts in mind can help you maintain optimism and a fighting spirit.

Psychological therapies—the "medicine that doesn't come in a bottle"—may be worth reviewing so you may pursue approaches that appeal to you (see Chapter 9). Counseling, alone or with a partner, may help get at how the illness has affected you and the one closest to you. Parents of young children, often concerned about what to tell their kids about their illness, need help in making these decisions.

When anxiety, insomnia, or depressed feelings get out of hand from dealing with treatment side effects or personal problems, it is important to seek help. Groups in which members in the same stage of illness share their feelings help a lot. Group members understand what you are going through as no one else can, and the networking with others is a big support. Most important is to keep in mind that you are not alone. Others are going through the same problems and are available to talk with you. You may learn to use relaxation and meditation in a group setting, which you can use later when you are alone.

For some, the uncertainty of the future brings about existential worries that lead many to seek solace from spiritual or religious sources. (This subject is discussed more fully in the following chapter.)

In summary, many tumors today recur or progress after their primary treatment, only to be successfully controlled for years by hormonal therapies, radiation, chemotherapy, or surgery. The dictum that recurrent cancer equals death is surely no longer true. Many cancers can be treated on a long-term basis so that they become chronic conditions. *Cure* may not be possible with today's knowledge, but effective *control* of the tumor, often for years, has changed the outlook. The human side becomes the challenge of how to live well with a chronic medical condition, how to continue to undergo treatment while maintaining the activities that are important in life, such as physical activity and work. Juggling all these elements, including helping your family to adapt to the changes, requires an emotional resiliency and maintaining a sense of hope.

14

THE LAST TABOO

I have Stage IV metastatic ovarian cancer. There is no Stage V.

—Vivian Bearing, the central character in *Wit,* a play by
Margaret Edson. Bearing is a professor of English and a
scholar of seventeenth-century poet John Donne

*Look, it's only death. It's not like losing your hair or
all your money. I don't have to live with this.*

—Harold Brodkey, author of *This Wild Darkness*, in
which he used humor to describe his advancing illness

*It is amazing, but I live with two diametrically opposed
views. On the one hand, I can't believe I'm going to
die, but on the other, I know I'm going to die. Make
some sense out of that!*

—Dorothy, a thirty-five-year-old artist
with metastatic sarcoma

*What do you say when someone asks, "How are
you?" when you're as sick as I am? I say, "I'm fine,
and my sister says I'm crazy."*

—Jenny, a businesswoman of fifty
with metastatic lung cancer

*It's not myself I'm worrying about. It's my mentally ill
daughter, who will be left alone without my wife or me
to look after her.*

—Bruce, a seventy-eight-year-old retired lawyer
with metastatic colon cancer

We all have to die sometime. I just happen to know a little more about how and when mine will be. It gives you time to plan and take care of things you want, to make sure you do certain things right and correct some things you would like to make different.

—Dominick, a seventy-five-year-old retired welder
with metastatic bladder cancer

My major concern is that I do this well. If I can, I will be a model for my children to remember. I hope it will make it easier for them when they face my situation.

—Martha, a sixty-five-year-old teacher and college
administrator with advanced uterine cancer

Most people die as they have lived; some with metaphysical and religious concerns on their minds, others, with the everyday preoccupations they have always had.

—Sir William Osler, eminent physician and medical
educator of the early twentieth century

I'm an absolutely confirmed atheist. Would you believe I found myself saying "God, help me," the other day. I don't get it."

—June, a sixty-year-old laboratory scientist with
Stage IV cervical cancer

$\mathcal{A}$ couple of years ago, my colleagues and I were asked to put together a conference for oncologists on psychological problems dealing with death. When we tried to think of a provocative title for the conference, we came up with "The Last Taboo." We realized that talking about the deeper meaning of life and death is still a taboo in American culture. Even today, we still feel uncomfortable and awkward talking about these kinds of issues. Sex, increasingly more explicitly shown in our society, has been lost long ago as a taboo, as we have been revealed as a nation of secret voyeurs.

Sex is no longer a taboo subject. In fact, almost no topic is held back from public display and discussion—except death. Death is something we want to forget about. A 1991 Gallup poll showed that Americans almost never think of death, or think of it only occasionally. Children are shielded from it at a personal level, though ironically, they are exposed by the media to its most violent aspects. Arnold Toynbee, in 1973, noted that in our society "death is considered un-American, an affront to every citizen's right to life, liberty and the pursuit of happiness." We live in a culture that extols rugged individualism and a philosophy of life that says you can accomplish anything you set your mind to. And we infer that includes beating out death. It is little wonder, then, that people are unprepared when an illness, like cancer, strikes with its potential threat of death. The result is a crisis of great proportions: One must confront not only biological death, but squarely what it means not to be alive. Dorothy, the young artist quoted at the beginning of this chapter, expressed this crisis of meaning so clearly when she struggled with the inability to imagine she could die, despite the intellectual awareness that her illness was not curable.

"What does it mean not to *be*?" "What is death?" "What does it mean to *me*?" These questions frame the existential crisis we all must face at some time. In this chapter, we deal with the human side of illness when death is the inevitable outcome. Treatment has changed, at this stage, from control of disease (discussed in the previous chapter) to treatment aimed at comfort, relief from pain and suffering, and maximal quality of life despite illness.

Dr. Jared Kass, of Lesley College, has cast this existential reality in a helpful light by calling it a *crisis of meaning*. This concept comes from the work of Viktor Frankl, the Viennese psychiatrist who wrote about the deeply human need to find meaning in life. Facing illness at an advanced stage creates a need to try to make some sense out of what is happening, to establish some coherence, which means to give it some meaning, to try to "get things back under control" as events tumble out of control. Daniel Callahan, Ph.D., eminent ethicist and author of *The Troubled Dream of Life,* feels that much of our present obsession about "death with dignity" is really a veiled attempt to *control* dying. What we are actually doing is finding ways to avoid the real issue, the meaning of death itself; death is still unthinkable and unspeakable.

Another aspect of illness that leads one to search for meaning is the sense of utter helplessness. "I feel so totally helpless in the face of this illness," people with advanced disease frequently say. Some people, aware of their personal helplessness, reach out for something stronger, more powerful than self. This leads many to recall the old belief systems that provided solace and a sense of connection to some more powerful figure, like God. The crisis of meaning is diminished by the ability to find some coherence, meaning, and connection to some greater whole than oneself. This is where the psychological and spiritual meet in the care of patients near the end of life.

In *palliative* care (care aimed at providing comfort and not focused on cure of disease), the crisis of meaning is embedded within four issues, broadly referred to as the pain and suffering associated with illness. They are:

- *The physical:* the experience of pain or other troublesome bodily symptoms

- *The psychological:* the emotional confrontation with your own death

- *The social:* facing separation from those you love most in life

- *The spiritual:* the need to reach out to a stronger, more powerful force beyond self, to a transcendent presence or connectedness

The Book of Job is probably our best source for understanding this type of pain and suffering, as Rabbi Harold Kushner points out in his book *When Bad Things Happen to Good People.* Job goes through overwhelming suffering with the loss of his family, his livelihood, and his health, as painful sores cover his body. The world's great religions all offer principles for dealing with suffering. Religious beliefs enhance coping by promoting a feeling of control and calmness despite the uncertainty, the threat of death, the frightening unknown, and the loss of all that is dear. They also provide a set of moral values and a model for behavior during periods of suffering. Prayer and meditation offer solace and comfort, and are available as a way to reach out at will to a higher power. What is important is an explicit existential perspective: a concept of life and death, of life after death, and of connection to a larger whole.

These concepts relate to a broad spiritual outlook. For some, this may be more philosophical than religious, but whatever the source, it yields meaning. The point is that we all have some well-honed beliefs, perhaps not well articulated, but nevertheless there to be called on during a crisis of meaning. Having a strong belief system and ties to others who share it gives you a leg up on the situation. Others have to struggle to find their own way. Callahan noted in 1995: "The meaning of death is . . . relegated to the privacy of religious beliefs or, in their absence, whatever personal resources people can bring to [it] on their own." You are pretty much on your own, since our society doesn't offer any "built-ins" to make it easier to talk with others to help find our own way.

This is when those of us who offer counseling can help you tap into your own resources. Our purpose is not to say "I have this great system to give you," but rather to assist you in sorting out your own beliefs that can help you. Viktor Frankl wrote: "The psychiatrist cannot show the patient *what* that meaning is, but he may well show him that there *is* a meaning, and that it remains meaningful under *any* condition." It is a personal journey, and a true helper is not one who asks you to change your beliefs but rather one who says, "I'm here to help you find your own meaning."

The interaction of the psychological and spiritual, two big components of human suffering, often cannot be fully separated in dealing with illness of great proportions. In fact, Kass speaks of a "psychospiritual" crisis of meaning, acknowledging in that way that the two *are* intertwined. Our group at Memorial is seeking a form of psychotherapy that simultaneously addresses these issues. Irvin Yalom, in his book *Existential Psychotherapy*, points out the inadequacy of Freud's psychodynamic psychotherapy, based on the id, ego, and superego, to deal with the issues around life-threatening illness and death. He notes that our most basic concerns, which are brought to the fore by illness, are our fears of death, isolation, and meaninglessness, and our recognition of the absence of ultimate control over our lives.

The concepts of Viktor Frankl, as I suggested earlier, are helpful in dealing with serious illness. In his book *The Doctor and the Soul,* he makes the observation that we all share an innate, deep desire to give as much meaning as possible to our life, to actualize as many values as possible. He refers to this profound, immeasurable need as the "will to meaning." This need extends even in the face of suffering:

> *Even a man who finds himself in great distress, in which neither activity nor creativity can bring value to life, nor experience give meaning to it—even such a man can still give his life a meaning by the way he faces his fate, his distress, by taking his unavoidable suffering upon himself. Life holds a meaning for each and every individual, and even more, it retains this meaning to his last breath. Life never ceases to have a meaning.*

The Doctor and the Soul, a manuscript Frankl wrote before going to the concentration camps, was taken from him while he was at Auschwitz, and he rewrote it after World War II. This process of reflection and new writing led to his developing a form of psychotherapy based on meaning, called logotherapy, described in *Man's Search for Meaning.* He noted that man is *pushed* by drives but *pulled* by meaning. One must make a conscious decision to pursue the meaning "to form a picture of man in his wholeness—which includes the spiritual (not to mean religious)." Frankl feels that meaning is strictly personal, not universal, that it is unique to each individual, and that you must find your own meaning, which is different from that of others.

Frankl's meaning-driven concepts are played out daily as I see individuals struggle to give some meaning to their situation. Martha, the teacher quoted at the beginning of this chapter, was seeking to give meaning to her dying by "doing it well" (I think she meant courageously), so that her children might recall their mother's example when their time comes to face their own death. Bruce, the man leaving a mentally ill daughter, found meaning by trying to find a way to secure care for his daughter.

One of the most poignant stories about trying to find meaning in a painful, intolerable situation comes from Father Tom McDonnell, first introduced in Chapter 9. He chose to work the night shift at Memorial because "that's when people need me most." In one of his morning reports to me, which he calls *News of the Night,* he recounted his visit in a hospital room where a young man's mother lay dying.

Marcos accompanied his mom from Venezuela. He came because he spoke English and his mom could not. Dad made the painful decision to stay at home to care for their other child, who was severely retarded. Marcos is twenty-one and was greatly admired by the nurses and staff, not only because he's an attractive and wonderful young man, but mostly because of his total commitment to his bedside vigil. Today, the doctors told him that there was nothing more that they could do for his mother and that he would have to make a decision as to whether or not treatment should end. He asked to see me; he wanted to know about the morality of stopping treatment. "Would it be murder?" he asked. We had a long talk and he described one of the most poignant "deals" I've ever heard negotiated with God. He told me, "This is the deal I've made with God. God, I'm all grown up and I can accept it if you have to take my mom. But this is what I want you to do if you have to take someone to heaven. You can take my mother, but you have to leave these two other mommas [patients he met here at Memorial], because their children are not yet grown up and they need their moms." I knew that I had just heard the ultimate in human generosity. Marcos came to understand through our talks that he wasn't murdering his mother by stopping treatment. And he found a remarkable way to give meaning to his impending loss by asking God to protect the mothers he had come to like.

Tuesdays with Morrie by Mitch Albom has remained on the *New York Times* bestseller list for many months. It gets to the heart of the search for meaning through the philosophy of Morrie Schwartz, retired professor of sociology. Morrie may be our contemporary equivalent of Viktor Frankl. Albom, a successful sportswriter, inadvertently learned of the serious illness of his beloved professor of sociology from his college days at Brandeis University. Morrie had developed amyotrophic lateral sclerosis (ALS), often called Lou Gehrig's disease. Mitch saw Ted Koppel interviewing him on TV about his illness. Albom phoned Schwartz and went to see him in Boston. It was a meaningful reconnection of the two. After that, he flew weekly for his Tuesday "class" with Morrie. The book came out of these meetings, a "final thesis." Albom wrote:

> *The last class of my old professor's life took place once a week in his house, by a window in his study where he could watch a small hibiscus plant shed its pink leaves. . . . the subject was* The Meaning of Life. *It was taught from experience. . . . No books were required, yet many topics were covered including love, work, community, family, aging, forgiveness, and finally death.*

Morrie recognized his special status and used it as a platform from which to talk about his situation, with great humor:

> *"You know, Mitch, now that I'm dying, I've become more interesting to people. . . . Here's the thing. People see me as a bridge. I'm not as alive as I used to be, but I'm not dead yet. I'm sort of . . . in between. I'm on the last great journey here—and people want me to tell them what to pack."*

And he did tell them, through Mitch:

> *"So many people walk around with a meaningless life. They seem half asleep even when they're busy doing things they think are important. This is because they're chasing the wrong things. The way you get meaning in your life is to devote yourself to loving others, devote yourself to your community around you, and devote*

yourself to creating something that gives you purpose and meaning.

"The truth is, Mitch," he said, "once you learn how to die, you learn how to live. You strip away all that stuff and focus on the essentials. Learn how to die and you learn how to live. . . . It's natural to die. . . . It's part of the deal we made. . . . The fact that we make such a big hullabaloo over it is all because we don't see ourselves as part of nature.

"We think because we're human we're something above nature. Now, here's the payoff. Here is how we are different from wonderful plants and animals. As long as we can love each other, and remember the feeling of love we had, we can die without ever really going away. All the love you created is still there. . . . You live on in the hearts of everyone you have touched and nurtured while you were here. . . . Death ends a life, not a relationship."

Morrie's courage comes through as another example of one who found meaning, even in battling the progressive symptoms of ALS.

I have found it hardest to write this chapter. It's much easier and more fun to write about survivors. It feels uncomfortable trying to express ideas and emotions relating to death. While this is challenging, it is also emotionally rewarding, because it forces me to look at life and death as a whole, that look we usually want to avoid. It isn't by chance that death and grief come so near the end of the book! It's hard to find the best words because we all face death quite differently, as uniquely as we have lived. Osler said it well, indeed, in 1906, as quoted at the beginning of this chapter: "Most people die as they have lived." If metaphysical and religious concerns are your thing, you use them, while for others, they die "with the everyday concerns they always had," that is, in their own unique way.

It is interesting to look back and see how this existential crisis has been handled by society in different ways at different times in the past. In the nineteenth century and well into the twentieth, one did not reveal the cancer diagnosis because of the prevailing attitude that cancer equaled death. It was considered cruel to take away a person's hope since the prognosis was zero. A "white lie" was justified to keep the ill person from knowing the truth. Of course, the patient was acutely aware of symptoms and signs of progressive illness, the reality of what was happening, but he or she also responded to the taboo by asking few questions. A facade of "everything's going to be okay" prevailed, with all parties recognizing the unspoken truth but with honest discussions occurring only between the doctor and family.

This isolation was described beautifully in Tolstoy's nineteenth-century story *The Death of Ivan Ilyich*. Ilyich, minister of the Court of Justice, falls ill with a pain in his side that does not improve; in fact, it grows worse. Yet his doctors and family pretend and make light of it. Tolstoy wrote: "This deception tortured him—their not wishing to admit what they all knew and what he knew, but wanting to lie to him concerning his terrible condition, and wishing and forcing him to participate in that lie." Tolstoy described the tremendous sense of isolation and loneliness of his character, knowing that he was getting sicker and sicker yet having those around him denying it. Only his servant Gerasim honestly acknowledged his illness. When Ivan Ilyich apologized for his helplessness, Gerasim said, "Oh, why sir, what's a little trouble? It's a case of illness with you, sir." And this decent act, Gerasim's reaching out to Ilyich and holding his legs in a comfortable position, is a kind of solace that *someone* acknowledges his reality.

The first papers published on patients' reactions to cancer, in the 1950s, from the Massachusetts General Hospital and Memorial, noted that patients asked fewer and fewer questions about their illness as it progressed. The patient acquiesced to the power of the conspiracy of silence, in which only doctor and family communicated honestly. Our notions of what is most kind and humane are sometimes misguided.

We owe a great deal to Dr. Elisabeth Kübler-Ross, who began writing in the 1960s to bring death "out of the closet." She started talking to dying patients in the 1950s and then began to speak and write, always passionately, about the fact that many patients *did* want to talk about their imminent death. She wrote a book, *On Death and Dying*, that was a powerful influence, particularly on nurses taking care of patients with cancer and also on patients themselves, who found it one of the few books available to read about serious illness. She pointed out in her latest book, *The Wheel of Life*:

Once patients started to speak—for some merely whispering was an enormous and taxing challenge—it was hard to get them to stop the flow of feelings they'd been forced to repress. Most said they had learned about their illness not from their doctors, but from a change in the behavior of their family and friends. Suddenly, there was a distance and a dishonesty, when what they wanted most was the truth. Most of them felt their nurses were more empathic and helpful than their doctors. I remember one woman crying out, "All my doctor wants to talk about is the size of my liver. What do I care, at this point, about the size of my liver? I have five children at home who need to be taken care of. That's what's killing me. And no one will talk to me about that!" With a chaplain's help, she was able to experience that most wanted honesty, closure, and peace.

Kübler-Ross influenced cancer care tremendously, at a time when disclosure of the diagnosis was increasing, anyway, based on the issue of patients' rights to knowledge of their illness and informed consent for treatment. This openness was useful, but it led staff to be more assertive in talking about death, and many patients who chose not to talk about it were forced to do so by well-meaning staff. Kübler-Ross also proposed that patients with cancer go through stages of dying, ending in acceptance. The stages, too, were overly interpreted. Some patients were considered "stuck" in a particular stage in going through the progressive psychological steps to acceptance. In actuality, I have encountered very few individuals who genuinely seemed to accept death as Kübler-Ross described. These concepts have been softened over the years, with a return to Osler's premise that we are each unique and "die as we lived." Hospice philosophy has changed to recognize people's inability to "do nothing" and wait to die. Trying a new treatment or a complementary therapy suggested by someone is far more the mode today, even while receiving hospice care.

At about the same time that Kübler-Ross was working in the United States, Dame Cicely Saunders began her groundbreaking work in London. Initially, she tried to get better treatment of pain for dying patients and, later, to improve the overall conditions for patients with incurable illness. The use of morphine was restricted to a set schedule, and she realized that many patients were suffering terrible pain because the morphine was not being given according to their level of pain and on a schedule to prevent pain from breaking through; pain was being treated only when it became severe. This was the beginning of the clinical study of pain control, which has changed patients' experiences and is beginning to reduce fears of "I'll be left to die in pain." These efforts led Dame Cicely to develop hospice care, which she established at St. Christopher's Hospital in London.

The first hospice in the United States was established in the 1960s in New Haven, Connecticut. Today, there are hospices in most cities. The hospice system encourages maintaining the person at home, if possible, bringing equipment and emotional support to the patient and family. This is far more readily achieved today, with pain medicines more easily given at home by means of infusion pumps, intravenous lines, and skin patches from which the analgesic is absorbed. Most people, when asked, say they would prefer to die at home. However, many also are concerned about the burden that is placed on the family. Sometimes, it simply isn't possible to keep the patient at home, and the hospice unit comes closest to being homelike, with its focus on caring.

The philosophy of care directed toward the physical, psychological, social, and spiritual aspects of illness is far more widely accepted today. There is still some reluctance on the part of families and patients who equate referral to a hospice program with abandonment and feel the medical caretakers have given up on them or their loved one. However, when they experience the hospice and its remarkably kind and understanding staff, they lose these concerns.

Ira Byock, a palliative care physician with great compassion, points out that the time near the end of life can be one of great emotional growth. I have seen families who seemed to experience some of their truly finest hours as they drew closer and were able to acknowledge both their love and their pain. Dame Cicely, in a recent lecture in New York, said, "I think it is a gift to be able to know what is coming and to allow one to use the time of living for doing and saying things that otherwise might remain unsaid, like 'I love you, I'm sorry, and good-bye.'" These last hours are far better spent in a quiet atmosphere than in busy hospital units geared to acute care.

People vary enormously in how much they can verbalize powerful emotions under the stress of advancing illness. Often the conversation is mundane, but both patients and loved ones know and feel the poignancy and profound reality of the moment. Those unspoken emotions are exchanged as truthfully and powerfully as if their farewells had been verbally expressed. Sometimes, the survivor feels guilty for not having said more, without recognizing that the dialogue followed the same pattern that characterized all their previous interactions. This is another instance of human communication for which there is no right or wrong way, only what feels right. I recall the time when my mother was very ill with colon cancer in rural Texas. Her communications about illness and death followed the pattern she knew from early in this century, perhaps also tempered by the Texas philosophy of seldom stating the obvious, especially if it is laden with emotion. We had only one conversation in which we talked about her cancer and her wishes about treatment. She did not want surgery and chose to "take my chances" and to remain at home. We both knew what this meant, but as she grew sicker, we never mentioned the word *cancer* or the outcome. It wasn't necessary to repeat the words for us to share the closeness of our moments together and the awareness that these were, indeed, last moments.

Terry Tempest Williams, in her remarkable book *Refuge,* carries the reader through her mother's illness and death. She points out the value of silence. After listening to the music of Chopin together, her mother says, "I just want to listen to the silence with you by my side." And she tells us of the importance of touching when her mother says, "It feels so good to hold your hand. I don't feel so disconnected."

We have been through a period recently, almost as bad as the "white lie" era, which has been dubbed the "truth-dumping" era, sometimes wryly called "terminal candor." Given the legal mandate to disclose the medical facts and prognosis, some doctors have found it easier and less emotionally draining simply to announce the facts and then leave the room. As Jack Price, who was quoted in an earlier chapter, put it, there is then no one "to pick up the pieces on the floor." Fortunately, this practice is being replaced with the availability of better training of doctors and the knowledge that it isn't so much what you say but how you say it. One can give painful news in a kind and compassionate manner, as discussed in Chapter 5, and encourage hope to attain realistic goals—not a cure, but the hope to visit a special person, for example, or to attend an important wedding or other occasion. We have to temper truth telling with allowance for hope to be maintained, even when this is formidable.

A remarkable play, *Wit*, received the Pulitzer Prize in 1999. Written by Margaret Edson, a kindergarten teacher in Atlanta, the play gets to the heart of some of the inhumanities of medical care through the voice of Vivian Bearing, a brilliant English professor and scholar of John Donne's sonnets. Bearing uses her wit (which means "wisdom" in its oldest sense) and humor to do intellectual and emotional battle with both ovarian cancer (putting it into a more tolerable context) and the physicians who typify all the "how not to's." This battle is aided by a nurse, who understands and advocates for Bearing. While the stage setting is sparse, Bearing, originally and superbly played by Kathleen Chalfant, fills the stage with her presence; she is barefoot and wearing a hospital gown and a red baseball cap to cover her baldness. The quote at the outset of this chapter—"I'm told I have Stage IV ovarian cancer, and there is no Stage V"—reflects the flavor of her jousting with the disease. She is equally acerbic with the doctors: "What do you do for exercise?" "Pace." "Are you having sexual relations?" "Not at the moment." This mix of humor and humanity, in a woman who has devoted her life as fully to seventeenth-century poetry as her physicians have to modern medicine, is a tour de force. A woman of singular purpose, Bearing finds solace in a friend, who comes to read to her in a tender exchange of affection as she nears death.

For some, like Vivian Bearing, hope is sustained—and is sustaining—in the face of overwhelming disease. Many who come to Memorial for a consultation choose to "fight to the end" and seek the newest, latest experimental treatments we have. Others find this kind of hope hard to understand and choose the comforting care of hospice.

Each is following his or her own usual pattern in reaching decisions.

Michael Lerner tells the story of his father's battle with cancer, which he fought to the end. Lerner is the director of Common-weal, a center for support services for cancer patients in Bolinas, California, and the author of *Choices in Healing*, in which he describes the range of alternative and complementary therapies. His father, Max Lerner, wrote *Wrestling with the Angel*, in which he described his passionate love of life.

Michael Lerner has a deep insight into the healing of spirit and psyche, which can take place when healing the body isn't possible. His interest was sparked by his father's battle with three cancers and death at eighty-nine of a stroke. Ironically, Michael says his father never pursued any of the therapies his son researched. His father coped by never giving up hope. Michael wrote in an article in *Reform Judaism*:

> Even in the face of what sometimes seemed unsurmountable odds and terrible suffering, he struggled on, nursing and protecting the hope that somehow he would survive. Was he reconciled to his dying? Not at all. He fought death every inch of the way. There was no consoling belief in a life after death. He fought because he believed that every wonderful thing about life was contained in the life we know: the life between birth and death.

My husband, James Holland, was Max Lerner's oncologist, and they shared many philosophical discussions between the "medical" parts of his visits. They also shared an optimism that sustained Max and likely has sustained Jim throughout his years of treating patients who are battling cancer. Michael observed:

> I have seen people days away from death who continued to hope for recovery and this hope was an essential element in coping with the ultimate life experience. I know many other cancer patients who were years away from death, who had no fear of death and some who even looked forward to death with curiosity, interest or relief. But although they had no difficulty accepting the prospect of death, they also had hopes: hope of a death without too

much suffering, hope of a death with dignity, hope of a death that did not impoverish the family, hope of a death that would reunite them with a husband or wife who had died before.

When we hope, we can heal. Healing is an inner process through which a person becomes whole. . . . The healing process has a tendency not only to bring people closer to appreciating their individuality and their unique purpose in this world, it also brings them closer to God, spirit, inner peace, connectedness or whatever we choose to call that which is great and mysterious.

We come full circle back to our search for meaning, even at this stage of life. Michael Lerner speaks clearly about the ways that people individually and successfully use hope, in different ways and with different meanings.

The opposite of hope, hopelessness, is a devastating emotion that saps the psyche in a profound way. It takes away energy, purpose, and the strength to interact with others at a time when this is so important. Hopelessness, along with depression, most characterizes the person who asks for physician-assisted suicide, seeing nothing left to hold on to or to "hope for." There is always hope, even when it is grounded in stark reality. It is possible to entertain two coexisting levels of awareness, one that intellectually recognizes "the reality" that the end of life may be nearing, and another in which a flicker of hope is kept alive by the inexorable advances in cancer treatments and by the benefits gained from the expanding range of alternative therapies.

Dr. Avery Weisman and his group at Massachusetts General Hospital also contributed to our understanding of the concerns that trouble patients with cancer. Through Project Omega, Weisman studied the distress of patients and their "existential plight." He identified those who were most vulnerable and defined those likely to be most in need of help. He, too, acknowledged that finding meaning was critical, along with proper handling of distress and symptoms and the maintenance of morale.

Project Death in America, established by the Soros Foundation, has had a profound influence on the culture around dying in America in the 1990s. Dr. Kathleen Foley, a physician at Memorial Sloan-Kettering who pioneered in the field of pain research, treatment, and palliative care, has directed this effort from the beginning with a tremendous impact. This concern for quality of life in the face of death has come at a time when the debate over rational suicide has focused attention on another aspect of end-of-life care: the right of the person to ask a physician for assistance with suicide. As contentious as the debate has been, it has led to public discussion of this important topic. My colleagues and I favor the availability of far better palliative and hospice care for all; we feel that physician-assisted suicide is a fast-answer cop-out to a complex problem. It glosses over the need for public and medical education about better end-of-life care. This care should be as aggressive at treating pain and suffering as the treatment that was aimed at cure.

One aspect of suffering is depression, which is in itself a high predictor of requests for physician-assisted suicide. Dr. Harvey Chochinov, a psychiatrist in Winnipeg, Canada, found that there are great day-to-day fluctuations in terminally ill patients' will to live and wishes for hastened death. These variations have to do with such factors as the severity of physical or psychological symptoms at a particular time and events in the family. The instability of the wish to hasten death suggests that patients who ask their physicians to help them die may feel differently later, if they have the chance. Some people assume that frail, elderly individuals would be the most positive about physician-assisted suicide. In a study by Dr. Harold Koenig and colleagues at Duke University, however, only 39 percent of elderly with chronic illness condoned physician-assisted suicide for terminally ill patients. Ironically, among their interviewed relatives, 59 percent favored the measure. It is interesting, also, that spouses and children were only marginally able to predict how their ill, elderly relatives would feel about the subject. This information suggests that living wills are important and that it is risky to make too many assumptions about how people who are most vulnerable feel about the legal initiatives.

The point to remember is that depression among these patients can often be relieved. We need to give more attention to improving medical care, as opposed to putting the emphasis on changing the laws. The diversion provided by Dr. Jack Kevorkian and his "suicide machine" has had the unfortunate effect of blurring the real issues.

Dr. Kevorkian has been hailed as a hero and protector of the dying. In fact, few know that he is a pathologist who never took care of a live patient in his medical career. He barely knew the patients whose suicides he assisted; he did not assess their pain and suffering (including treatable depression) prior to arriving at his decisions to help them carry out their suicidal wishes.

The U.S. Supreme Court's decision to allow state-by-state action on this issue has been wise. The Oregon experience so far has been thoughtful. Other states have not jumped to get on the bandwagon; it is wise to engage in longer deliberations about this issue.

A recent study of people receiving dialysis for kidney failure or AIDS, done by Dr. Peter Singer in Toronto, gets closer to what patients consider most important in their end-of-life care. While no cancer patients were part of this study, the findings show what very sick people want during their care at the end of their life. First, patients wanted to be sure their pain and other distressing symptoms were going to be controlled. Constant, unremitting pain is intolerable, and it *can* be controlled today with only rare exceptions. Unfortunately, the public needs more education to reduce these fears. Continued education of doctors and medical students is also needed to ensure they know how to use all the new analgesic agents and procedures.

Other symptoms can be as distressing as pain: shortness of breath, anxiety, inability to eat or sleep normally, diarrhea, and nausea and vomiting are common ones. With good palliative care, these symptoms can be controlled. Many research trials today are testing ways to control each of these symptoms. Too often in the past, such symptoms might have been dismissed as "going with the territory." Not so today in palliative care, which is improving at a fast rate. In fact, the first Chair of Palliative Medicine in the United States was established in 1998 at the Albert Einstein College of Medicine with the appointment of Dr. Russell Portenoy, signifying a new level of recognition in medicine of the importance of this aspect of care. The control of physical symptoms and psychological distress must be the focus of care. These issues are important not only for the patient, but also for the family members who look on and observe. Family members often have indelible memories of loved ones who suffered without relief. These memories become part of their grieving and complicate the burden of grief (see Chapters 15 and 16).

Another finding of Singer's study was that people feared being left "lingering," kept alive on machines with no hope of getting better. They did not want to be left as a "vegetable" in a prolonged dying process. They also wanted to ensure they would be a part of the decisions made about their care, or else that their chosen proxy would make the decisions. This concern reflected a need for a measure of control over their situation, a respect for their wishes. They wanted to avoid being a burden on their families to the extent possible, for example, by making a living will dictating their wishes for care so that relatives would not have the burden of making decisions without knowing what they wanted. The organization Choice in Dying has information about living wills, including the laws of each state (www.choices.org). Having the document helps, but a frank talk with whomever you choose as your health proxy is equally essential.

The patients in the study wanted to strengthen family relations by talking openly about their situation, even though it was uncomfortable and often had to be done when the opportunity arose. Family members are often overwhelmed and upset by such talk and avoid it, sometimes out of fear of saying the wrong thing and sometimes out of the wish to bolt. The areas of concern to patients studied by Singer and his colleagues about end-of-life care have at their core the need to respect each individual's wishes to be free of intolerable symptoms.

Following is a discussion of the major concerns patients with terminal illness want addressed in their care at the end of life.

CONTROL OF PAIN AND SUFFERING

Intolerable pain leads to hopelessness and giving up. I have a dictum for our staff that we cannot evaluate a person's anxiety or depressed mood until his or her pain is controlled. When that is done, the mood often changes for the better and anxiety goes down. I recall an elderly Chinese man with an advanced cancer of the neck who was brought in by his children because of a suicide attempt. He had been unable to communicate his distress to them about the terrible pain in his throat from the cancer. When his pain was controlled in the hospital, his ability to cope returned. His family was grateful to be able to reunite with him, with a renewed purpose: to insist on his telling them when he had pain at home so that it could be treated.

Anxiety can be disabling, and it is common in people who have shortness of breath or uncontrolled pain. Panic attacks and anxiety with restlessness, inability to go to sleep or stay asleep, jitteriness, and racing heart are all treatable and should not be considered things that must be tolerated without relief. Medications can control anxiety at this stage of illness without causing drowsiness. Being awake to interact with the family is important; many patients admonish me: "I don't want to be zonked and not able to talk with my visitors." Many people also like to practice relaxation techniques or meditation, which may bring them a sense of peace and tranquillity (see Chapter 9).

The stigma of psychiatric care arises again in the area of palliative care: Patient and family are concerned: "Why are you asking a psychiatrist to help?" They feel it is somehow disrespectful of the person who is ill. ("Of course he's depressed; what do you expect?" or "You're just going to knock him out.") They don't understand that a psychiatrist can play an important role in the treatment of the forms of distress with which oncologists and generalists are sometimes less familiar. This role involves, in part, providing support for you and your family, but also recommending medications as needed. Medications can reduce extreme anxiety and panic and leave you more comfortable and calmer to cope better. Similarly, the tremendous fatigue and drowsiness that pain medicines cause can be decreased by stimulants that can help you feel more alert and able to undertake meaningful tasks during the day.

Finding the right bedtime medication to ensure sleep is important also. These symptoms, as well as depression and confusion, are treatable, and with their control, you can be more like your usual self, to the great relief of your family (see Chapter 9).

Depression has been discussed as well as its troublesome counterpart, hopelessness. I trust we have made it clear that hope should never be given up or that one should never feel there is a time when nothing more can be done. It is important for people to realize that comfort is an integral part of treatment, and it should be approached with full vigor. The debate concerning physician-assisted suicide hinges in part on whether physicians are willing and able to recognize and treat depression. The concept that it is "normal" at this stage to be depressed and that there is no treatment for it is wrong. Yes, it is normal to be sad, but true depression is something else: It is the sense of isolation with no ability to enjoy even a simple thing, an extreme fatigue, a mood that stays "down" no matter what, inability to eat or sleep, and hopelessness with a wish to die or to receive help with suicide. These symptoms of depression need careful evaluation and treatment (see Chapter 9).

HELP IN FINDING MEANING

The meaning that you derive in your ordinary healthy days will likely affect the way that you choose to spend your time during even a serious illness. I am impressed by how helpful it is to so many patients to be encouraged to focus on completing a piece of work that is important to them. Many physicians who are accustomed to a vigorous daily schedule find solace in directing their energies toward a paper or research study that must be completed. In the same way, work becomes a vehicle for feeling productive despite illness, a way to remain a part of a professional community, and a way to leave a legacy by contributing to a familiar area.

Another effective strategy that helps many people is to ask them to review the important aspects of their lives. Often I hear, "But I've done nothing important. I made no contribution to the world." However, when I look back with them, they share with me recollections of special relationships, of their impact on a friend or child, or some special achievement that reflected altruism. Morrie Schwartz said it well with, "People die, but not relationships. You live on in the hearts of others." By reframing their lives, patients gain a new perspective that leads them to see the difference they have made in the lives of others. The life narrative approach provides a way to view your life from another vantage point, one that sees the broader picture, the meaning of a life lived.

Psychotherapy can be yet another vehicle in the search for meaning at this stage of life. Now it is directed toward finding out, first, your concerns (about death, the dying process, the anticipated separation from loved ones, and the impact on family members). Part of the existential distress is recognition of leaving all that life means and all those one loves. This causes intense mourning of the loss that is coming. Acknowledging and expressing these feelings is comforting both for the patient and for the family. Separating the grief surrounding these losses from depression is important. Depression represents an added burden that can complicate the ability to cope with grief and the emotions that often surface; depression adds feelings of guilt, worthlessness, suicidal despair, and the inability to enjoy any activity. Supportive psychotherapy can give you emotional assistance with these problems, is responsive to your changing needs, and can help you to have greater awareness of your strengths throughout life.

Susan Block, of Boston, noted in a report to the American College of Physicians:

> *Psychological distress is a major cause of suffering. It impairs capacity for pleasure, meaning and connection in the present, erodes quality of life and amplifies pain and other symptoms, reduces the ability to do the emotional work of separating and saying good bye, and causes anguish and worry in family and friends.*

Yet distress still remains underrecognized and undertreated.

Father Tom McDonnell uses an interesting analogy, which works well with children and some adults as well, to give a tolerable meaning to pain and suffering. It combines the psychological and spiritual in a unique way.

> *Living near the beach, I've gotten into the habit of collecting ocean-washed stones as I walk my dog. I've often used a stone with*

children to encourage them. I call them my "don't be afraid stones." I ask the children to listen to the story of the stone: "Let the stone tell you about the earthquakes and the thunderstorms and the moving earth plates and the fierce storms that brought it to where it is now. It used to be much larger, it used to be a different shape altogether. Along the way, it had many challenges and scary times. Look how they've smoothed it down to where it fits in the palm of your hand. Feel how far it's come, and it's not finished yet. In fact, it was on its way to the beach when I picked it up and asked it to help you get through this rough time. It'll help you."

The stones help adults, too:

Ellen, a woman with ovarian cancer, was considered one of the most difficult patients on the floor. She had massive pain that wasn't well controlled, and her distress often came out as anger with the staff. I was asked to see her. Our first encounter seemed hopeless, and she invited me to "get the hell out of my room." On my way out, I asked her if she would mind if I kept her in my prayers and asked God to help her with all this awful pain. Her entire disposition softened, and she gently asked how prayer could possibly help, and even if it could, how could she possibly pray in all this pain? I returned to her bedside and we explored the possibilities of joining her anger and her pain and throwing them both up at God as the best possible prayer we could come up with at the moment, given the NOW we seemed to be stuck in. As we talked and prayed it became obvious that fear was among the worst parts of being sick— fear for herself, her daughter, and their future.

I had one of my "don't be afraid stones" in my pocket. I gave it to her with my "listen-to-the-story" line. She cried and smiled very gently. Gathering stones had been her hobby for years, and she took it as a certain sign that we should be friends. In every one of our subsequent visits, the stones were part of our conversation.

Janet was another severely ill woman for whom the "don't be afraid stone" became a source of comfort. She suffered from advanced-stage lung cancer, and panic attacks were fairly common when she

*began to experience oxygen deprivation. She took to the stone imme-
diately and would tell me stories of the stone's adventures, a device by
which she was able to tell me her story. She was fond of clutching the
stone as she napped, and one day it was lost . . . someone cleaning
had simply thrown it out. We resolved the loss by agreeing that the
stone was still on its way to the beach somewhere, just like ourselves,
and along the way it just got "trashed." Needless to say, the Atlantic
Ocean provided still another "don't be afraid stone."*

Father Tom is one of those pastoral counselors who are powerful with patients because they combine the spiritual with the earthy
mundane, and often with good humor, to help people cope. He is a
highly skilled pastoral counselor for patients with severe illness.

The Reverend George Handzo, director of the Chaplaincy Service at Memorial, has compiled a list of the most common problems
people bring to him and his chaplains: isolation from religious community, grief, guilt, hopelessness, concerns about death and afterlife,
conflicted or challenged belief systems, loss of faith, concerns with
meaning and purpose of life, concerns about relationship with deity,
conflict between religious beliefs and recommended treatment, and
ritual needs.

The Gallup poll mentioned earlier found that people, while
healthy, say they would like clergy to be available if they became
seriously ill to provide spiritual support and to deal with concerns
about death, what comes after death, feelings of guilt, distance from
their faith community, and concerns that illness is punishment.

STRENGTHENING TIES

Concern for the closeness of others when one is ill comes up over
and over; it only increases with the advancing level of illness. A
Gallup poll showed that this is especially true of younger people:
They felt it important, in the face of severe illness, to have someone
with whom they could share their fears and concerns and who could
hold their hand.

The threat to these ties is a part of the existential crisis of illness. How does one talk about the unspeakable? I have had several young couples come in to talk about how they should tell their children about the illness of one of them which could end with death. One father stands out in my mind:

Philip was a successful lawyer whose life with his wife and young children was suddenly shattered by his diagnosis of colon cancer that had spread to several sites, including the liver. Unfortunately, his chemotherapy treatment did not shrink the tumors. He and his wife came in seeking advice on when and how much he should tell his six-year-old son and four-year-old daughter. We discussed the fact that children need to feel "in the loop." Otherwise, they sense something is wrong, but not knowing what, many assume they caused the problem or that things are much worse than they actually are. Philip's concerns were for his wife and the children to a far greater extent than for himself. He had lost his own father in childhood and knew the pain it had caused him. He was particularly concerned for his six-year-old son, Charles, who could better understand what was happening. He wanted some way to tell his son he would always be with him in spirit. They had seen the movie *The Lion King* together, and it provided him with a way. As he is dying, Mufasa, Simba's father, talks with Simba, pointing to the night sky, and says in effect, "When you look up at night and see those twinkling stars, you know I am there watching over you." Philip used this story to give his son the message of his own love and continuing presence.

Other movies and books are useful in preparing children, such as *The Land Before Time,* a film in which the mother of a baby dinosaur dies and he must find his way, but she returns in his thoughts to guide him when he is in trouble. (See Resources at the end of the book for additional reading.)

. . .

In summary, with both children and adults, the last taboo, that unspeakable topic, is part of the tapestry of life. We do better if we can openly discuss it and put it into a perspective that gives some meaning to life and death. As we have explored in this chapter, there are many ways of finding meaning: psychological, spiritual, philosophical. Any and all of these ways should be respected and encouraged. People at the end of life have a right to a broad approach that gives them full care for all their needs: attending to their distressing physical and psychological problems, helping them to strengthen their ties to others, and ensuring that their spiritual needs are met. Such an approach to care must incorporate a team of people who share the philosophy of hospice care that addresses all these dimensions. We are coming closer to meeting these needs, but much remains to be done in training doctors, medical students, and nurses. Patients and their families can contribute by pointing out their need for this type of care and by influencing public policy. My fervent hope is that one day soon, exploring the meaning of life and death will no longer be taboo.

THE FAMILY AND CANCER

I feel like the woman in the movies who is tied to a rail-road track and the train is barreling down the track, getting closer and closer.

> —Josephine, whose husband was being
> treated for pancreatic cancer.

There's an elephant sitting in the room and nobody's talking about it.

> —Roberto, whose elderly mother tried to protect her
> children by not talking about her colon cancer

People call all day long asking how Debbie is doing. Nobody ever calls to ask how I'm doing.

> —Jane, Debbie's partner of fifteen years

*I*n a way, it is hard to talk with you about the specific ways cancer impacts on the family because there are so many different constellations of families with differing relationships. You may be the spouse or life partner of a loved one who is seriously ill; you may be the child, parent, sibling, or close friend. Sometimes, a grandchild, niece or nephew, or daughter-in-law becomes the primary caregiver for the person who is ill. Each of these relationships raises unique issues. For example, older parents caring for their ill adult child fear the loss of their child. A life-threatening illness in a child triggers an overwhelming sense of injustice in the parents. The well spouses or partners now must juggle most or all of the family responsibilities—household, finances, child care, work—while caring for their ill loved one. Adult children may find it hard to put their own lives on hold while taking care of an ailing parent.

Discussing family issues that apply broadly is further compounded by the need to take into account a family's ethnic origin, cultural values, religion, and attitudes toward illness. This requires careful and sensitive attention. In today's world, there is greater diversity in the makeup of the nuclear family. Gay and lesbian couples represent an increasing number of households. Also, it is important to keep in mind that not everyone has a family when illness strikes, especially not older people, for whom friends may become surrogate families.

Despite these acknowledged differences, some universals still apply. The overriding question is: How do you deal emotionally and physically as a caregiver, not only performing your usual tasks in the family, but shouldering new responsibilities that are strange and unfamiliar? As caregiver you have multiple roles to assume in relation to supporting the patient. In a large study sponsored by the United Hospital Fund in New York, Carole Levine used focus groups to obtain data from a range of caregivers. Her report gives credence to the importance of caregivers. Information in the following sections is based, in part, on this report.

THE CAREGIVER AS TRUSTED COMPANION

Little thought is given by the health care team to how hard it is to assume the role of trusted companion for an ill loved one. You must be outwardly empathic and supportive of the patient, while inside you are feeling heartbroken, having trouble controlling your emotional pain and despair. In studies of caregivers, about a third have significant distress, believing that they should have help for *their own* symptoms. For example, mothers of children who have gone through bone marrow transplants continue to have anxiety, depressed mood, vivid recall of the treatment, and dread that it could be needed again. These worries continue long after the child has recovered physically.

So it is important, as you set out to help your loved one along the cancer journey, to build in your own support system, which will ultimately benefit you both. Asking family members and friends to pitch in to give you a breather goes a long way and prevents you from becoming overwhelmed. You must feel able to cope yourself to be able to support your loved one. Counselors are available who are familiar with the patient's illness, for example social workers on the oncologist's team. Inquire at visits to the oncologist about resources for yourself. If the social worker is unable to help you, he or she will refer you to someone who can.

A forgotten participant in the illness may well be the child or children at home. They need to be monitored for how they are coping and, if needed, referred for counseling. Nowadays, more groups exist for kids who have an ill parent.

Like many caregivers, you may be part of the cancer journey "from the beginning," starting with the concern about a physical symptom that may be cancer and the office visit, when the diagnosis and treatment plan are presented by the doctor. It is important to listen carefully to be able to reflect later on what was said (see Chapter 5) and to help the patient make important decisions. It is crucial to be there to give support and comfort if the news is bad. Your presence alone can make it easier for your loved one to hear bad news. Telling this special person in your life that "you don't have to face this alone; I'll be with you every step of the way" can be reassuring to the point of making the "impossible" seem possible. The simple task of accompanying the patient to treatment means driving or arranging transportation or missing work or personal appointments, but because it is absolutely necessary, it gets done.

Caregiving is often a balancing act between the psychological and the logistical. Besides giving emotional support, you may need to schedule appointments, pay medical bills, handle insurance, keep track of medications, and keep family and friends informed of the status of the treatment. It can be helpful to appoint another family member or friend to serve as an information clearinghouse for family and friends. You keep that one person informed, and everyone calls her or him. This simple arrangement frees you up to deal with the person who needs you most at this critical time. Your exact role will likely depend on how you and your loved one work together on problems. Couples who work together as a team will find it a frequent occurrence to turn to each other, asking "What should I do?"

Decisions about embarking on or changing a treatment plan need input from another person. The trusted companion role means reflecting on the options, considering them, and helping the loved one come to a decision. The more serious the decision, the harder this is. You must determine whether more information is needed, such as a second or third opinion. You as companion often must explore Internet resources, call the National Cancer Institute (1-800-4-CANCER), or call the American Cancer Society (1-800-ACS-2345) to get more information. Your loved one is likely to be upset, and too much information may increase his or her anxiety. You can serve as a helpful filter for the raw information, which is part of being the trusted companion.

This role can cause conflict with some doctors, who respect the patient's autonomy and may be suspicious of the trusted companion as an intruder in the dialogue. Yet the reality is that few of us make important decisions totally alone. In our focus groups with doctors, they noted that patients often consulted their families when considering treatment on a clinical trial: "If the families are positive about a trial, it is likely the patient will agree. The families' and friends' influence on the decision is unquestionably very strong."

Your role as companion becomes more difficult when your loved one is admitted to the hospital. "Being there" becomes critical to maintaining your loved one's morale and providing a familiar presence. Levine points out that the family feels the need to be present out of a sense of loyalty and feels guilty if not present, which may not be understood by the medical staff. Intensive care units can be trying for the trusted companion, since the level of illness is high and visiting hours are often severely limited. Staff can be supportive of the caregiver, but their attitude can turn sour when they feel pressed too much by a caregiver who insists on remaining at the bedside. Some staff aren't comfortable with the family watching the mechanics of care in the intensive care unit, genuinely feeling it only adds to the patient's distress and to the family's as well.

It is practical, during care in the intensive care unit, to appoint one family member to deal with the doctor and nursing staff, if possible. Large families should try to take turns visiting to avoid overwhelming the hospital staff and exhausting the patient.

When the patient is a child and the caregiver is a parent, the need to "be there" becomes even greater. We normally want to protect children from harm, and when illness strikes we feel the pain and guilt (even if irrational) of not having been able to protect them. As Karen Swymer, the lawyer, mentioned in Chapter 11, who was treated for sarcoma at the age of eleven, recalls her mother saying, "If I could do this for you I would." One parent usually has to give up working when a child is treated for leukemia or one of the other serious childhood cancers. Being present as a buffer to the world of hospitals and clinics is a major role that provides reassurance and security to the child. Disruptions at home, including having less attention to give to siblings, cause additional guilt and problems. The need for the parent to control his or her emotions and be able to give emotional support to the child is a tall order: managing pain medicines and being watchful for changes that foretell worsening, while thinking about whether the child will survive or not: "Can I stand it? What can I do? How do I best comfort him?"

THE CAREGIVER AS ADVOCATE

The family caregiver has a delicate but essential role as advocate for the patient, which can put him or her at odds with the medical staff. When the ill person is fully alert and assertive by nature, the family member's role as advocate is minimal. But when the person is seriously ill, is a child or a frail elderly person, has a language barrier, or is cognitively impaired, the family member becomes the central link to the care, the interpreter of the patient's needs, and the person who feels responsible to ensure that the care given is appropriate. This role can be difficult and stressful, especially if the situation is colored by a prior negative hospital experience. In these situations you feel that you must be vigilant to ensure that the care is proper and attentive. The tension with the hospital staff can become intense if the staff members interpret your questions and concerns as distrust or criticism, and they may fail to understand your role as advocate.

Most hospitals today have a Patient Representative's Office where you can voice complaints and receive a rapid review of the problem. This innovation has provided support for families, as a supplement to the traditional first-line support of social workers.

A similar situation can occur in an office visit. When a patient is too ill to keep up with medications, the caregiver must attend the visits to clarify the medicines taken at home and on which schedule. It is best to bring in the bottles of medicine and to report details to the doctor that the patient may forget. Make notes of the doctor's instructions concerning medications and signs that a problem may be occurring. Ask for a written daily calendar of what should be taken morning, noon, or night, or on an hourly schedule.

In the focus groups we did with patients and family caregivers, both spoke about how helpful it was when family members were welcomed in the doctor's office. Patients liked it when the doctor knew family members by name and asked about children or those absent. One patient said: "They have always said, 'Have the family come in.' There are times when it is so crowded in those little clinic rooms that it looks like a Marx brothers movie. But I feel my family can ask questions, and we get the information we want."

Not everyone finds it so easy to get the information needed. Rhonda Price, whose husband Jack was treated for an advanced melanoma, told a group of physicians: "My job is in management, so I see my situation as caregiver spouse as a management problem. I'm managing Jack's illness, my family, my child care, and my work. The only way I can do this is if the doctors and nurses give me the information I need to do my job."

Today, e-mail is a helpful resource you may be able to use for rapid communication with your doctors. Finding a time when you can speak with your doctor on the telephone is often frustrating, but e-mail allows for sending and receiving messages at will.

In our focus groups about doctor–patient communication, one particularly sensitive physician spoke about attending to family members' emotional needs:

> *I find just sitting there with the family and just providing some*
> *support and letting them express their fears or letting them cry, or*

whatever, that seems to help. You really cannot take away the disappointment and sometimes there is not much you can actually say. Just being there, or just being quiet, is enough. Your presence with them seems to be helpful. Sometimes, I find in these situations that saying nothing is better than saying something.

I am reminded of David Spiegel's paraphrase of the old admonition "Don't just stand there, do something." He says, "Don't just do something, stand there." There are times when less is truly more.

The role of advocate, like the role in decision making, can be complicated by problems in the family that relate to prior conflicts originating long before the onset of cancer. Dr. Marguerite Lederberg, a psychiatrist in my group and well known for her work with families and the ethics of care, feels that a critical intervention is calling a meeting of family members, patient, and key staff to clarify problems and conflicts that would otherwise simmer and grow worse under the stress of the increasing severity of illness. Such a meeting serves as a way to identify a dysfunctional family member or pattern of interaction so that counseling can be offered to ease the situation and provide longer-term help.

At times, the family wants information kept from the patient. Often this is because the family members have trouble handling it and project these difficulties onto the patient. I have seen this with adult children of elderly patients who insist, "Don't tell Father, he won't be able to take it." Yet when I speak to the father, he might say, "Of course I know it's cancer, but my children can't accept it. They feel better thinking I don't know." Sometimes, I see the reverse situation: A patient doesn't want the family to know the diagnosis. This is hard for the doctor, who wants to respect the patient's rights about disclosure but feels the diagnosis would be better shared. Many physicians get around this problem by insisting on talking to the patient and family together so that they all hear the same information at the same time, can ask questions, and can discuss it among themselves afterward.

Views about revealing or withholding the diagnosis are powerfully influenced by culture, and providers must be sensitive to the origins of the requests (see Chapter 5). We often have patients from

Russia or Eastern Europe, where revealing the diagnosis and prognosis is still uncommon. As a family member you may have to explain to the doctor that telling the diagnosis to a patient is considered cruel in your culture, and try to arrive at a solution that you and the doctor feel comfortable with.

THE FAMILY MEMBER AS HOME CAREGIVER

Current health care policies require hospitals to discharge patients "sicker and quicker," solely on the basis of the economics of managed care, thus making families an indispensable, but formally invisible, piece of health care. In the United States, there are now about 22.4 million families caring for their chronically ill loved ones at home, underscoring the public health problem that this represents. Today, you are expected to provide not only the emotional support expected of families for millennia, but also a remarkable range of services, including the use of high-tech equipment that we would have believed not possible a decade ago, assuming that only highly trained professionals could handle that level of technology. Not only must you assume this responsibility, but you may be given little instruction on how to do so. Under these circumstances, it is perfectly normal to have enormous anxiety about whether you might be doing harm. It becomes crucial that you have a good line of communication with your loved one's physician. This may be through a nurse who is the frontline person and available by telephone; her close work with the doctor ensures you have access when you need it.

Carole Levine's study showed that "more than 25 million family caregivers are struggling with the fragmented, inflexible, and increasingly complicated collection of institutions and agencies called 'the health care system.'" A recent survey by the American Association of Retired Persons (AARP) estimated that one in four households in the United States is involved in family caregiving. Levine says, "It sometimes takes a cross between heroism and martyrdom to survive as primary caregiver today." You may feel some of both on some days. This issue has not yet been addressed at a federal level, and caregivers often function without benefit of technical or psychological support from medical and social agencies. There remains little quality control and oversight of home care services; economic gain has frequently been a higher incentive than quality of services rendered.

Clearly the benefits of care at home weigh in heavily against the liabilities. The patient is in his or her own private world of familiar walls, furniture, and bed. Friends may come and go; there is a feeling of greater independence. The benefits for the family are daily, informal interactions; more control of care; and a sense of satisfaction and pleasure at being able to provide care for a beloved family member or friend.

However, home care is not best for every patient or every family. Studies of palliative care are showing evidence of "caregiver burden," the stress that can be put on families when they care for ill relatives at home. These obligations are superimposed on ordinary responsibilities. As a caregiver, you must:

1. *Maintain the stability of the home and family.* This includes attending to the daily tasks of meals, household chores, arranging for child care, and other normal activities in addition to caregiving.

2. *Ensure family income is maintained.* Depending on the level of care the patient requires, you may need to quit your job or take leave from work to provide care for the ill person at home. Employers vary in their tolerance and support for work leave or absences; however, research suggests that overall income goes down when someone in the family is seriously ill. Reduced income and extra costs take a toll on funds available for other family needs, like children's schools and saving for college education. According to the AARP report, caregivers' out-of-pocket expenses related to groceries, medicines, and care-related costs average $171 per month, which is an estimated nation-

wide expenditure of $1.5 billion per month, or $18 billion per year. The economic value of informal (unpaid) caregiving, if it were reimbursed, would be astronomical—18 percent of total national health care spending.

3. *Seek the services of a part-time or full-time companion or aide.* The cost of a full-time paid caregiver at home varies from $25,000 to $50,000 per year, restricting their availability to families with higher incomes. Medicare currently supports four hours per day, three days per week, for a home health aide. Even hospice care provides only twenty hours per week of care. In homes with lower incomes and limited resources, the burden usually falls to mothers or adult daughters, many of whom have small children and who also work. The AARP survey found a higher percentage of homes with a chronically ill family member among minority, underserved families.

4. *Manage the patient's physical care.* As discussed earlier, families must now provide much of the patient's physical care at home. Studies have shown that this is extremely stressful for the family caregiver, who must meet the demands of nursing care without having any medical or nursing skills or training. Discharge planning at hospitals is often done at the last minute, without adequate instructions or training in how to manage equipment or give medication. Rhonda Price, Jack Price's wife, highlighted this problem for me, pointing out that medical staff often aren't aware of what they ask of the family. She remembered that once Jack was discharged during a change of nursing shifts. Rhonda said, "I'm double-parked in front of the hospital to pick up my husband.

I'm trying to deal with taking him home, and
nobody on the floor knows what's going on or
can tell me what he will need at home." Discharge
planning, with instruction of the patient and family about what to expect at home, is fine in concept, but it doesn't always work out the way it was
intended.

The symptom that causes the most stress is pain. The caregiver is
anguished at seeing a loved one in pain and yet is fearful of giving
too much medication, fearing it could hasten death. This dilemma
is agonizing for the family, and it is a frequent reason for rehospital-
ization. Managing intravenous lines or catheters, oxygen, and the
patient-controlled analgesic (PCA) pump can be overwhelming.
Shortness of breath and anxiety are disturbing and frightening.

Dr. Sherry Schachter, a nurse, psychologist, and grief counselor
at Memorial Hospital who has specialized in home care, notes that
the level of physical exhaustion of the caregiver correlates with the
level of illness of the patient. She feels families underestimate the toll
taken by the physical care, such as keeping the bedclothes and room
clean, dealing with the mountains of daily laundry, making special
foods that appeal or are required by a certain kind of diet (or that can
be eaten easily by their loved one), and staying up with the patient
during sleepless nights, often with little support. It is little wonder
that the feeling of being alone with the problem is so common.

5. *Tolerate the "medicalization" of home.* The good news
   is that a broad array of "high-tech" equipment can
   now be brought into your home to control symptoms. IV fluids for hydration, total parenteral
   nutrition (TPN), pumps for pain control, special
   beds, devices to move the patient from bed to
   chair, oxygen inhalation—all these contribute to
   making the patient far more comfortable at home.
   The bad news, however, is that, in a sense, you
   have been invaded by the hospital's moving into
   your home. The sanctuary you call home now

contains foreign objects and a flow of individuals
from outside who must monitor the equipment to
keep it working. The much-appreciated intimacy
you looked forward to on getting your loved one
home becomes constrained by these forces.

One wife whom Sherry Schachter came to know in our Home
Support Program was pleased to have her husband's care at home.
Her husband had a twenty-four-hour nurse, a feeding tube, an intravenous line for antibiotics, and an infusion pump for receiving anal-
gesics. However, she felt totally excluded from the bedroom, which
she called their "Mini-ICU," and she mourned the loss of the
chance to share closeness with her husband in the remaining time
they had together, which she had wanted so much.

Carol Levine, herself a caregiver to a chronically disabled spouse,
voiced the problem this way:

> *Professionals call us "informal caregivers" to distinguish us
> from paid workers, implying that there is something casual and
> nonessential about our care. Because we love the people we take care
> of, we do not ordinarily see ourselves as anything but a spouse,
> child, sibling, partner, friend. In fact, we take care of the basic
> health, social, and emotional needs of people who are disabled or
> chronically or terminally ill, and who are only sporadically
> hospitalized. Sometimes, we have to turn our homes into something
> like small hospitals, crowded with high-tech equipment.*

Attention to the problem of home care could prevent hospitalizations and nursing home placement. The United Hospital Fund
report noted several changes that could make a difference:

- Discharge planning should be made a process, not a sin-
  gle-shot event, with better training of families for the
  tasks they must do at home. Better education and communication with staff in the hospital and continued contact at home with medical staff would be invaluable.

• Support programs should be made available for caregivers including counseling, general support, and respite sources (substitute caregivers for brief periods). When the caregivers surveyed by Levine were asked what they wanted for themselves, they answered: "Someone to talk to who understands what I'm going through." "Someone to call when I have a question." "A day off." "A kind word from a doctor, nurse, or social worker." According to the AARP survey, when caregivers were asked how they coped, they responded they used prayer (74 percent), talking with friends (66 percent), exercise (38 percent), and hobbies (36 percent).

• Accountability needs to be established for quality of home care services.

There is a great need for national attention to the plight of families of the chronically ill. Some pilot efforts are occurring in some states to provide compensation for the care given at home, recognizing that this "invisible" part of health care is buckling without help. Some experts contend that if families stopped providing care, the health care apparatus in this country would collapse. Tax breaks, additional home health aide hours, respite care, and other initiatives by the federal government are needed to address the problem.

As illness brings new roles, each family forms it own internal, implicit agenda, assigning roles to each member. Tasks include earning a living, attending to household chores, caring for the children, and setting the social agenda. Illness turns the status quo upside down. Often the breadwinner can't work, and either must struggle with the new role of being ill, dependent, and cared for by the other partner, or with putting work on hold to provide care. Or the caregiver must now become the breadwinner in addition to performing his or her normal tasks. And the caregiver feels it is important not to show anger at the added role so that the ill person does not feel guilty. The delicate balance tips at times, and frustrations and conflicts erupt.

Children may not get the affection and attention they need and normally would get. They feel anger, fear, and guilt that they may have contributed to the family's current situation in some way. They may be fearful not only that the ill parent will die, but also that they may eventually be abandoned if anything happens to the well parent. School performance often plummets, behavioral problems arise, and the well-being of all family members is disrupted. Often, members of the extended family, when available, join the household to fill in the gaps in services. Grandparents may be pressed into service at a time when they are ill-equipped to take on responsibilities of child care. Intergenerational conflicts may appear in the context of illness. The world of health is replaced by that of illness, and it affects the dynamics of the whole family. The more serious and chronic the illness and the more uncertain the outcome, the greater is the disruption for all.

Advanced and chronic illnesses also mean greater involvement with the health care team. In a strange way, relations with the doctor, nurse, and social worker, especially if the patient is a child or adolescent, become so important that these professionals become like an appendage of the family. Their reactions and their views of how things are going each day become yardsticks of "how we're doing."

When illness abates and treatment ends, roles must change again, and that can stir up trouble as well. The ill person roars back to show renewed health and vigor, proudly saying, "I'm a survivor"—to the horror of those who have watched through the illness and fear a relapse. Caregivers may become fearful and angry that the sacrifices they have made will be squandered in the effort of the new "expatient" to too rapidly regain a normal life. They may try to overprotect and keep the survivor under wraps longer than is necessary.

At the same time, well family members may fall into the new roles so completely that they don't welcome losing them. Strains again arise as a new equilibrium is sought. Counseling for the family can help them sort out what has happened. Dr. Jamie Ostroff, psychologist, and Dr. Peter Steinglass, child and family psychiatrist, have found it helpful to bring several families together to discuss their problems jointly after their adolescents' cancer treatment is over. Parents talk together while the adolescents meet alone, and then they all meet together. Sharing experiences and hearing one another's solutions has proved helpful for recovering the health of the family after illness. This approach places the illness in the larger context of the families' lifelong experiences. It becomes part of the family myths and stories: "what it was like when Joanie was sick."

THE FAMILY AND GENETIC RISK

Dealing with genetic risk is a new aspect of a family's psychological burden that has emerged in the last decade. The family is concerned that its well members will develop the same cancer as the one who is ill due to a higher genetic risk. You have probably heard of BRCA1 and BRCA2, genetic mutations that increase the risk of breast and ovarian cancer. Women who develop breast cancer often immediately begin to feel guilty and anxious that they have put their daughters at risk. They have the double worry of their own breast cancer and the possibility of their daughters' developing it. In point of fact, the proportion of new breast cancer cases each year with a genetic origin amounts to about 5 percent; however, the information has been so widely circulated, especially as genetic testing has become available, that women whose relatives have breast cancer are highly fearful about developing the disease. They often say, "I'm a walking time bomb. It's only a matter of time." Fortunately, genetic testing usually reduces anxiety because women's imagined risk generally exceeds their actual risk. In general, close surveillance through a special clinic or by a vigilant gynecologist is adequate for care.

Genetic counseling and testing for BRCA1 and BRCA2 are available today to clarify for a woman whether or not she is a carrier. BRCA1 carries primarily a breast cancer risk. Women are often advised to take Tamoxifen, which reduces breast cancer risk. Removal of both breasts as a preventive measure is drastic and is rarely recommended. BRCA2 carries the risk of both breast and ovarian cancer. Removal of the ovaries may be recommended when the risk of ovarian cancer appears high.

The genetic information, whether it is positive or negative, is often helpful in resolving the uncertainty. Testing positive (when the genetic marker is found) permits closer surveillance by mammography, clinical examination, and breast self-examination to pick up the earliest signs of disease. It also is a call to alert daughters to begin mammograms at an earlier age. Psychologist Dr. Kathryn Kash has counseled these women and found that group therapy, in which those at risk share their fears and their coping techniques, reduces anxiety. It is important to control their anxiety since Kash found that those who had the highest anxiety had trouble doing their breast self-examinations and getting mammograms.

Colon cancer also clusters in families. One familial form has a high frequency of developing at young ages. Genetic counseling is essential. The more common form of genetic risk is handled by regular colonoscopies to identify polyps, the removal of which prevents the development of colon cancer. Families with a history of colon cancer need to make their members aware of it and begin colonoscopies at an early age.

It appears that prostate cancer also carries a genetic risk, and regular digital examinations and PSA testing should begin by age forty in men in these families.

Genetic testing for cancer is a rapidly developing field. Use your knowledge of your own family history to guide you in cancer surveillance to ensure early diagnosis of any cancer that might develop. Be sure also to adopt the healthy habits outlined in Chapter 12, which apply to everyone. Genetic testing will likely become more common, but at present it carries several liabilities. First, results are often inconclusive. The second liability relates to health and life insurance. Information that should be kept fully confidential can sometimes be found out, including the fact that a person took a genetic screening test. A positive test can lead to discrimination in obtaining medical insurance.

From a psychological perspective, people have tolerated hearing results without serious problems. When one person in a family is tested and found positive, the issue arises of informing other family members and suggesting that they be counseled and tested. Family conflicts can ensue when there are differences in opinion about the value and appropriateness of testing.

WHAT IS POSITIVE ABOUT BEING A CAREGIVER?

Our knowledge of the stresses and difficulty in coping has largely focused on the negative side of home caregiving. But there is a strong positive side to being a caregiver for a loved one who is ill. In a study of partners, one of whom had AIDS and one of whom was the caregiver, psychologist Dr. Susan Folkman showed that good feelings coexist with the sad, painful feelings. Even while going through the extreme stress of caring for a critically ill partner, caregivers felt a deep sense of closeness that was engendered by providing hour-by-hour physical care. They also felt the satisfaction of being able to show love in this way. The same picture emerges when the caregiver is a family member or friend of the patient with cancer. "As hard as it is, I wouldn't have it any other way" is a frequent expression. The awareness that "I've done all I could do" helps alleviate the normal pain and guilt that accompany grief after loss. Positive feelings accompany the effort to improve the patient's comfort, despite the illness.

In exploring this issue, Folkman asked the caregivers: "Tell me something that happened that made you feel good, that was meaningful to you and helped you get through the day." Virtually all the participants could clearly recall positive events that occurred in the midst of the severe illness of the partner. The events were ordinary, like a dinner, a word of appreciation from another, going to a movie. One recalled looking at a beautiful flower in a street stand and noticing how it stood out in an instant flash, creating a special moment for both. What made these ordinary events special was that the caregivers felt more connected and cared about, and they felt good about themselves and what they had done. It was an emotional "breather" from the daily chores.

The underlying theme of having coexisting positive and negative thoughts and emotions was the search to find meaning in the face of all the negatives inherent in the situation. The meaning varied for the men studied. Spiritual and religious beliefs were a source of positive meanings, especially beliefs of reunion after death or some comforting and peaceful understanding of death. The negative feelings of distress were sprinkled heavily with positive ones, contributing to the overall sense of a "job well done."

This search for meaning is a task for family and friends and especially the primary caregiver of a person with cancer. They experience the cancer illness of a loved one with a range of emotions and activities, including empathy, comforting as much as possible, sharing decisions, being advocates, and providing physical and emotional care. Despite role changes, stresses, and distress, the positive feelings of "being there when it counts" and the sense of doing all one can for a loved one more than outweigh the stress of caregiving.

HOW DO I GO ON?

Hearts heal faster from surgery than from loss.

—Ellen Goodman, *Boston Globe*, January 4, 1998

She died, and the person I was died, too.

—A widower of seventy, following his wife's death

Life must go on; I forget just why.

—From "Lament" by Edna St. Vincent Millay

Remember me, when you can't go on;
Think of me, when all hope is gone.
When you're all alone and no one seems to care,
I will always be there.
For I am everywhere, and I have always been here;
Since time began, I am.
And I will never leave you, for I am your friend.
Just look inside your heart, take my hand.

—"Remember Me," lyrics and music
by JoAnna Burns-Miller, 1999

Grief is an integral part of our human condition. All of us have lost or will lose someone we love beyond all telling. Our social nature makes us want to bond and become attached to others. "'Tis better to have loved and lost, than never to have loved at all." For how many centuries has this saying been a guiding insight into our human relationships? Grief is the price of those attachments of love that we make in our lives. How we deal with it has a lot to do with how we can put the loss into a broader perspective that allows us to continue to live despite the engulfing void in our lives.

Grief demands expression of powerful emotions. We need an opportunity to tell and retell events, stories, and memories, all of these but reflections of our deep love for the person who has died. This is why it is so much harder when you have no one to talk with about how you are feeling. It's also true that some people are more vulnerable than others in the throes of bereavement and have more trouble overcoming their grief.

This book, devoted to the human side of cancer, is at its heart about loss, the threatened or actual loss of health and life. But it is also about surviving the loss of a beloved person who has died of cancer: spouse, parent, child, sibling, friend. "How do I go on after losing someone whom I loved so deeply and who meant so much in my life?" I hear this asked, sadly, all too many times. One in four families is touched by cancer. Indeed, cancer has become the leading cause of death in this country as heart disease vs. cancer mortality has diminished. This chapter describes the pain of grief and of the bereavement that follows the death of someone close.

Those who have experienced a significant loss and struggled to go on will recognize all too easily the feelings and emotions brought on by grief; I hope the discussion and suggestions for coping will be helpful. For those who have not yet been touched by loss, the chapter may not seem so relevant. But for readers who have a loved one who is ill and whose life is threatened by cancer, this chapter describes the feelings of grief, what is known about the human process of grieving, and offers some approaches that may help.

PATTERNS OF GRIEVING

GRIEF BEFORE LOSS

Death from cancer is often preceded by a lengthy period in which both the person who is ill and the healthy caregiver recognize the likely fatal outcome, while at the same time trying to deny it. This period is sometimes called a time of *anticipatory grieving*. However, no matter how clear the outcome is, and how prepared one believes one is, the actual death somehow comes as a surprise: "I didn't expect it so soon." "I was still hoping for the best." "I can't believe it's really happened."

GRIEF AFTER LOSS

The first hours and even days after the death are often recalled later as: "I was in a daze; I can't even remember it." "I was so numb I had no feeling at all." "I went through the funeral without even realizing what was happening." "It felt so unreal, as if I was watching a movie." "For days, my heart felt like a piece of stone." This is a kind of benign temporary denial of the painful information as the psyche tries to absorb the catastrophic information.

But the numbness is interspersed, in this acute stage, with waves of intense grief, of crying and sobbing, that come on several times a day, occasioned by a sympathetic word, a hug of affection from a friend who understands, or seeing some object that suddenly brings back the gravity of the loss. Caught up in a wave of grief, you become distraught, crying without easy control, and overwhelmed for a period of minutes with trouble regaining emotional control. Sudden vivid memories come back, coupled with a sense of unreality, disbelief, and panic, swelling to an overwhelming feeling that "I just can't go on." These waves are so difficult to bear that you try hard to prevent them by avoiding contact with people. However, the act of sharing the loss with another, as painful as it is, is actually helpful because it encourages talking about the loved one and sharing memories, which makes the loss real and reduces the feeling of "maybe it isn't so." It also celebrates the life of your loved one.

A panicky, anxious feeling accompanies the sadness and helplessness and makes it hard, if not impossible, to carry out daily tasks. You may find yourself wandering aimlessly around a room picking up objects without thinking or pacing in agitation with the thought, "I can't live like this." You may avoid activities that brought you pleasure before, particularly those that remind you of your loved one. For example, you may not want to listen to music that was previously a shared source of enjoyment because it makes you feel sadder. These feelings are all intensified during the waves of overwhelming grief described above.

Along with psychological distress, grief disrupts normal physical function. The abrupt change in your pattern of living—caused by the absence of a key person in your life—disrupts brain and biological rhythms (the body's normal twenty-four-hour rhythm of function), especially of the nervous, hormonal, immune, and cardiovascular systems. These physiological changes lead to the common physical symptoms of grief. For example, it may be impossible for you to concentrate, to keep your attention on any topic. Sighing respirations are common, and choking sensations occur often with crying. You may feel weak and profoundly fatigued. Sleep may be difficult, ranging from fitful to impossible. Food has little taste; it "sticks" in your throat. Weight loss is common, and you may look pale and ill, in addition to looking profoundly sad. Strikingly, many of these physical consequences seen in human beings are similar to reactions observed in animals. For example, Dr. Myron Hofer, a psychiatrist and researcher, has witnessed similar effects in infant mice when their mother is taken away from them.

During this stage of acute disorganization, you may feel distant from others and want to be alone. Yet you must go through the cultural rituals that follow a death: the wake, sitting shivah, the funeral, and the burial or cremation. These rituals around death developed over the centuries for a good reason: They counter the tendency to isolate oneself. They ensure that you are surrounded by others who care and who share the loss. For several days, you may rarely be left alone by family and friends, who wish to give you comfort with sympathetic words and gestures.

This complex picture usually persists for about six weeks. Dr. Erich Lindemann, chairman of Psychiatry at Massachusetts General Hospital in the 1950s and with whom I studied, carried out the first study of normal grief. In 1941, a tragic fire in the Coconut Grove nightclub in Boston trapped about five hundred young people inside. Most died or were badly burned. As the staff of local hospitals attempted to give medical care and comfort to the survivors and families, Lindemann documented the survivors' symptoms, their grieving, and its outcome. He found that after six weeks, the aimless, disorganized days and nights with preoccupying thoughts of the deceased, including hearing them speak or seeing them in a fleeting dream or dreamlike state, began to diminish. A more normal pattern of daily activity began to ensue. However, there was a wide variation in timing, in severity of symptoms, and in recovery.

This study was followed by those of many other outstanding researchers, who told us that we have held a lot of myths about grief that just aren't true:

1. MYTH: Grief should be over in a year.
   FACT: Grief lasts much longer than a year for many people.

2. MYTH: Grief goes through stages to final acceptance.
   FACT: There are no stages of grief and, often, no acceptance of the loss.

3. MYTH: Life should go back to normal.
   FACT: There is no "recovering" what is gone for many, but simply carrying on with a radically altered experience of life.

We know that when grief befalls a parent after the death of a child, or a spouse after the loss of a mate of many years, particularly after a long illness, there is apt to be prolonged grieving, and the loss is never fully over. Unquestionably, the death of a child is viewed as the most painful loss: "I've lost not only my child, but my future." For many people, the loss of one's mate or partner is equally traumatic. And then there are the losses made all the harder by a long-standing pattern of interdependence, such as sometimes exists between spouses, between parent and adult child, and between siblings.

I saw Mary after her husband of forty-nine years died of prostate cancer. They had a very close relationship and had woven a pattern of shared responsibilities typical of fifty years ago. She took care of the home and had raised the children, and he was the breadwinner and keeper of their finances. She participated little in these areas because it didn't seem important. During his illness, Bill tried to tell Mary about their financial affairs and to show her what she would have to do when the time came for her to take over these matters. She refused to listen. In the final months of his illness, Mary took total care of Bill, and this took all of her time. She gave up seeing her friends, and her only social contacts were telephone calls and visits from the children and grandchildren.

Mary found Bill's death hard to believe at first. She went through the religious services without showing great emotion and accepting comfort from others. The reality of the loss did not hit until her friends and children left, and she was finally at home alone. She became preoccupied with thoughts about Bill's illness and worried that she hadn't done enough. She ate poorly, did not want to cook, and lost weight. She cried all the time. Her family became concerned about a possible suicide risk when she told her daughter, "I really don't want to live. I'd rather join him in the cemetery now." At her daughter's insistence, Mary agreed to accept help.

Sessions over six weeks were devoted to her going over and over the events of Bill's illness and death, and her concerns about the last moments: "Maybe, if I had called the doctor a day earlier, he might have lived a while longer." She felt guilty that she hadn't done enough. It was difficult for her to let go of these feelings and recall the happy memories of Bill and of their long life together. When she talked about her concerns with her children, they tried to help by saying, "Stop talking about it. It's only making you feel worse." The effect of their response was to isolate her even more.

As we continued to discuss her loss, Mary was able to eat and sleep better and to socialize some. One year after Bill died, she was functioning better and had found an accountant to manage her affairs. However, she was still grieving and living much of the time preoccupied with memories of her life with Bill. Special family parties were so painful that she wanted to avoid them; however, for the sake of the children, who very much wanted their mother to be with them, she forced herself to go. She did take up the game of bridge again, and reconnected with her old friends. She attended a group for widows who shared their similar feelings. A year and a half after Bill's death, Mary realized that life would never be the same, but at least she now felt she could continue to live.

Grief Following an Unexpected Death

While cancer is a disease in which people often have time to prepare for a loss and to say good-bye, that isn't always the case. Sometimes there is no time for either the person who is ill or the loved ones to absorb what is taking place in a whirlwind of overwhelming medical problems and failed treatments.

Hans was a diplomat in his seventies, happily married to a woman twenty years his junior. He had carefully planned how his wife would manage when he died first. Neither he nor his wife was prepared for her diagnosis of acute leukemia, which did not respond at all to treatment. They both struggled with the reality, but the time was too short to grasp fully the true nature of her fatal decline before her untimely death a month later.

Hans was devastated and required help from friends to organize her funeral and burial back in Germany. On his return to the United States, he still could not believe his wife had died. "I imagine she is away on a trip." His grief was acute, and he cried and paced aimlessly for days. Unable to go out with friends, he stayed at home and went over and over the monthlong illness and what else might have been done. He tortured himself for not seeking an experimental therapy in Boston. Friends encouraged him to come to see me.

We talked at length about the enormity of his loss. He had had a clinical depression twenty years earlier, and after three months, we agreed he might benefit from medication.

He also agreed, reluctantly, to join Dr. Sherry Schachter's grief support group for people who have lost a loved one to cancer. In the group, he was able to talk more easily with people who understood his loss. Over the next two years his outlook improved.

GRIEVING OVER YEARS

The American way . . . has turned grieving into a set process with rules, stages, and of course, deadlines. We have, in essence, tried to make a science of grief, to tuck messy emotions under neat clinical labels—like "survivor guilt" or "detachment."

So whatever our national passion for emotional efficiency, for quality-time parents and one-minute managers, there are simply no one-minute mourners.

—Ellen Goodman, *Boston Globe,* January 4, 1998

The myth exists in our culture that there is an acceptable time period to be set aside for grieving, usually one year. But this ignores the reality of human nature. Each person is unique; each loss is unique. The expectation of a "deadline" beyond which you no longer grieve is just plain wrong and adds to your burden. This amounts to blaming the person who is grieving for his or her suffering, rather than trying to understand it—another form of "blaming the victim."

Parents know full well that they will never "get over" the death of their child. They hold the memories far too dear to let go. Life does go on for them, but in an entirely different way. I was honored to speak at a meeting of the organization In Loving Memory, which is dedicated to providing comfort and support for parents who have lost their only child or all their children. Over two hundred people gathered for this remarkable meeting in Vienna, Virginia, and shared memories of their children with others who knew exactly how they felt. Each wore pictures of their children, shared memories, and listened to discussions of the many facets of grief. It felt like a celebration of their children's lives, in a setting that made this possible. Many parents are still grieving years later, and some never fully recover or "put the past behind them."

In 1998, I took part in a TV segment on *20/20* about grief. The personal story of Rob, a young man whose father had died of cancer ten years earlier when he was a teenager, touched me.

> Rob and his family were interviewed on the day of his graduation from medical school. The day itself was bittersweet because it would have meant so much to his father, and the celebration was clouded by his absence. Rob tells of how earlier feelings of loss returned, for him and his family, on that graduation day, although it was a full decade later. He said that, for him, grieving was the only way of holding on to his father. Painful, yes, but also evidence that the tie was unbroken and that his father still was in their hearts.

There are similarities between the myth that there are stages in grieving (from denial to acceptance) and the notion that patients pass through psychological stages in their experience of a cancer illness. All the stages *may* occur during grief, but not in a set sequence and surely not in a way that leads us truly to accept the death of someone who was an intimate part of our life.

DIMENSIONS OF GRIEF

How we grieve, like how we confront a serious illness, is influenced by the attitudes of the society at large, as well as those of our own personal traditions. We see over and over at Memorial that people from certain ethnic groups are apt to be more demonstrative in their grief. The other extreme is the "stiff upper lip" that is expected in some cultures in which it is considered a sign of weakness to cry or show emotions in public, no matter how distraught one is. These attitudes and expectations can cause us to suffer in silence. We can feel like we're "doing it all wrong," when in fact there is no right way.

Social attitudes often differ among families regarding talking about death with young people. Children and teenagers have many questions, like "Where do people go when they die?" Some families answer the question by saying, "Grandma is in heaven" or "with God" or "alive in your heart and memory and feelings." It is often best to speak to children about death as straightforwardly as you can, within the context of your own beliefs and traditions, to help them to go on.

Several emotions that accompany grieving are important because they can come as a surprise. If you are prepared for them to arise, they may be easier to deal with.

GUILT

A major part of grief in its early stages is an obsession with the last days of the illness and "why" it happened, as illustrated earlier by the experience of Mary. Thoughts go around and around as you look for ways things might have been different, might not have ended in death. "What else could I have done?" "Did I make a mistake?" "Why did I go home that last night and not stay at the hospital?" "Did I take him to the wrong hospital?" "Did the doctor make a mistake?"

Vivid memories of the last days come back repeatedly, such as how your loved one looked, so pale and ill, sometimes in pain. People say, "Why can't I just remember the good days and forget the last horrible ones? But I can't get beyond how she looked that last week." This preoccupation with wanting to clarify the details of the illness and the causes of death often is connected with the feelings of self-blame and guilt, that somehow you could have done better or even have saved the person you mourn.

The present method of delivering health care contributes to this dilemma in a new way. When a person becomes critically ill, it often becomes important to know whether or not the patient wants to be resuscitated in the event breathing or the heart stops. In the absence of an advance directive in which the ill person has indicated his or her wishes in this regard, the next of kin or health proxy—usually a spouse or partner, a parent, an adult child, or a sibling—must be asked whether the patient is to be resuscitated. The decision to resuscitate may lead to the patient's being placed on a respirator with continued discomfort and pain; this decision may prolong dying.

Sometimes, saying no (Do Not Resuscitate [DNR]) makes people feel they are making the decision to give up, even while recognizing it as the wisest choice and one that the patient would have wanted. Not many of us would opt to prolong the dying process. But the more one loves the person who is dying, the harder it is to agree to "pull the plug." When Marcos had to resolve this question for his mother, he asked Father Tom (see Chapter 14), "Would it be murder?" Making this decision can carry an expensive price tag. Memories of it may come back to you during your grieving as another reason for guilt. The memories of how you made up your mind, along with your ambivalence about whether it was the right thing to do, may become a source of guilt that can complicate getting past the last illness.

> Jordan, a thirty-year-old husband and parent, signed the DNR order for his father, who had advanced colon cancer. Ten years later, he said: "I know it was what my father wanted, but it's still the hardest thing I've ever done."

Guilt also appears during grieving, for having survived—for being alive when the person you loved so much has died. I recall a mother who could not allow herself to smile or laugh because her son couldn't do that anymore, and she felt it would be wrong if she did. It took months for her to feel it was all right to laugh and take pleasure in life again.

RELIEF

Another common feeling is one of relief that the person, after a long illness, is past his or her suffering: "At least, he is now at peace." This feeling is accompanied by a newfound sense of relief for yourself now that you no longer have to watch the suffering, witness the daily painful ordeal. This sense of relief is strengthened for many by spiritual or religious beliefs. Most of us find this feeling completely rational and understandable. However, the sense of relief makes some people feel guilty, even though it is a reflection of reality.

ANGER

The other side of the guilt coin is anger. "If it wasn't my fault he died, then it had to be somebody else's!" Anger often turns to the doctor, nurse, or hospital; all become suspect, especially if the relationship at the end was not positive and trusting. Asking for an appointment with the doctor after the patient's death, to discuss the final events and the cause of death or to review the autopsy findings, can lay some of the worrisome questions to rest.

Usually, however, the anger is really about the absence of the person you loved; that person is no longer sharing your life. You know that he or she didn't want to have cancer, but in an irrational way you feel angry with the person for leaving you. This anger may be acted out by being irritable with others as they try to help.

ANXIETY AND HELPLESSNESS

The immediate feeling is "I can't deal with this; I can't make it alone." "I have never felt so alone and vulnerable before." You have a deep sense of uncertainty about how you will be able to tolerate the future on your own. Naturally, the death of someone extremely close to you prompts you to have thoughts about your own mortality. Thoughts of death, usually carefully tucked away, surface when someone close to us dies. We get a sudden stark look at our own mortality. This is especially true with the loss of both parents. As long as they are alive, we sense that "I'm okay because my parents will die before me." But when that protection is gone, our own vulnerability to death becomes much more real.

WHY DID IT HAPPEN?

This question gets asked over and over, particularly when the death is that of a child whose life was just beginning. We try hard to make sense out of it, but it just doesn't work. We believe in fairness and justice, but this event represents neither. We view ourselves as being moral, "good" people; why, therefore, should it happen to *us*? One of the most widely read books about this aspect of grief is by Rabbi Harold Kushner, *When Bad Things Happen to Good People.* Kushner's son died as a teenager of a rare progressive disease. He expresses this feeling of unfairness and chooses to honor Aaron's life by seeking to distill a blessing out of his pain and tears, in the hope that the book will help others who experience such an enormous loss:

> *I felt a deep, aching sense of unfairness. It didn't make sense. I had been a good person. I tried to do what was right in the sight of God. . . . How could this be happening to my family? If God existed, if He was minimally fair, let alone loving and forgiving, how could He do this to me? . . .*
>
> *I wanted to write a book that could be given to a person who has been hurt by life—by death, illness or injury, by rejection and disappointment—and who knows in his heart that if there is justice in the world, he deserves better. . . . If you want to believe in God's goodness and fairness, but find it hard because of the things that have happened to you and to people you care about, and, if this book helps you do that, then I will have succeeded in distilling some blessing out of Aaron's pain and tears. . . . His life made it possible and . . . his death made it necessary.*

Feelings of despair at the injustice and unfairness of the death of the person you love are often coupled with difficulty in sustaining personal faith in a God who can be viewed as loving. Yet that faith and firm belief are of great value to the many who believe. This was poignantly expressed in an inscription found on a retaining wall of a building in a concentration camp liberated by Allied forces in World War II:

> *I believe in the sun, even when it doesn't shine.*
>
> *I believe in love, even when I don't feel it.*
>
> *I believe in God, even when He is silent.*

TRYING TO MAKE SENSE OF IT

I discussed, in Chapter 14, Viktor Frankl's work and the need we have to try to make sense out of something that is senseless. Dr. Susan Folkman, a psychologist whose work we've previously mentioned, has studied individuals' search for meaning as a way of coping with the death of someone close. Folkman points out that when we have to face something like the loss of a cherished person, we first try to approach it as we ordinarily do, namely, to see it as a problem and solve it. But when we confront this particular problem, there is no solution, no way to "fix it." We try going over the feelings of loss again and again, only to return to the same dilemma: You can't fix it. It's like banging your head against the same wall over and over again, and nothing happens except you get a bloody head. John Bowlby, another early researcher in grief, described this repeated searching for the lost one, which is followed by despair when the person isn't found.

When the psyche can't change something, it resorts to trying to figure out how to view the loss in a tolerable context, to "make some sense of it." Being able to view the loss from a religious or spiritual perspective is helpful for those with strongly held beliefs. This may mean feeling close to the person who has died, by feeling a spiritual presence, and by a hope to be reunited in a future life. Searching for a transcendent meaning beyond the bounds of physical life provides a strong support during grieving. According to Folkman, we seek a larger, "global meaning." We must place loss into some larger perspective that is tolerable and that changes its meaning. "He must have died for some purpose." "It fits some plan that we don't understand." "It's God's will." This serves as a way to give an acceptable meaning to a senseless loss. Dr. John Spinetta, a psychologist, found that parents who had lost a child to cancer were helped when they could give some meaning to their loss.

COMPLICATED GRIEF

I have discussed the normal grieving process and how myths about it lead to inappropriate expectations. Sometimes, however, grieving is complicated by factors that make it much harder, some of which are outlined below. Most people with these issues can benefit from professional evaluation and treatment.

EFFECTS OF CHILDHOOD EXPERIENCES

Our view of the world and the goals, values, and expectations we adopt for ourselves have a lot to do with childhood experiences. If the world we grew up in was largely benevolent, with only the reasonable and expected troubles of childhood, we are more likely to be optimistic as adults, expecting good things from the world. On the other hand, when childhood has not been characterized by benevolence, when there has been physical or psychological abuse, we are, as adults, less trusting of the world, more pessimistic, and more suspicious of the motives of others. Many people manage to overcome these problems and, as adults, appear secure and well adjusted. However, when a person has had earlier, traumatic experiences, the loss of someone close can lead to an intense recall of the traumatic events from long ago, which compound grief with symptoms of posttraumatic stress. Grief is complicated by increased anxiety, fears, and helplessness. These individuals are vulnerable to additional problems during grieving.

Jorge was a man who sat by his young wife's bedside throughout her long course of ovarian cancer. When she died, he was devastated and found he could not bear to go on, even though he was aware that their children needed him. He was overcome with grief, and he had anxiety and frightening nightmares along with his profound sadness. When we talked, it was clear that Jorge had had a remarkably good marriage after he came to the United States as a young man. He had put his childhood in Puerto Rico behind him, never talking about it to anyone. It was as if his life began with his marriage. As we talked, Jorge described a childhood of physical abuse leading to his running away and coming to New York. The grief over the loss of his wife led to his inability to keep the buried traumas from the past out of his consciousness. Jorge could not prevent the memories from coming back in nightmares. He felt "weird," helpless, and confused that this was happening as he mourned his wife. "Am I crazy?" he asked. We met several times, and he began to take an antianxiety medication. He was able to connect his past with the present and to motivate himself to care for his teenage children, whom he wanted to protect from what he had experienced. Jorge talked through his enormous loss, how his life had been totally changed by his wife's presence and how hard it was for him to go on.

PROLONGED GRIEF LEADING TO DEPRESSION

At times, the symptoms of acute grief remain so severe that they simply don't improve at all. The lack of enjoyment of things that brought you pleasure in the past, along with sadness, isolation, and crying, begin to resemble the symptoms of clinical depression. Certainly, symptoms of depression and grieving overlap, and it is not always easy to tell them apart. Professional evaluation is needed to determine when severe grieving, that is, prolonged or unresolved grief, has become a clinical depression.

CUMULATIVE LOSSES

The idea that "we all have a breaking point" is surely apparent when people have a double loss, such as losing a spouse and a child in close proximity. This double tragedy is catastrophic, taxing the powers of making sense of it and adapting to a totally altered life. If the spouse was a breadwinner, the grieving person may also experience financial losses and the need to live with diminished resources. Depression following multiple losses is a common occurrence.

PHOBIAS AND FEARS

When a child dies in the family, the siblings have memories of the loss, but they also experience the parents' grief and fears for their safety. Parents may become overprotective, afraid of every minor symptom that occurs in their healthy children. The result can be to sensitize the child about vulnerability to illness. We sometimes see this reaction in adults who have excessive fears and phobias of illness, appearing to stem from their parents' response to the death of a child and their fears about illness of their remaining children.

EARLIER PSYCHOLOGICAL PROBLEMS

If you have experienced significant psychological problems in the past, you are vulnerable to more severe grief. If you had a problem with alcohol or drugs in the past, you should be alert to avoid using them as a crutch. If you have been seriously depressed, you are vulnerable to the return of depression. Recognizing your vulnerability is important so that you seek help early.

COMPLICATED FEELINGS TOWARD THE PERSON WHO DIED

At times, death comes to a person who had caused pain and anger to others. A son or daughter might never have resolved feelings toward a difficult father. A surviving spouse may have had a marital life that was a mix between affection and hostility. On the surface, it would appear that these circumstances should make grieving easier since there was less attachment. But it doesn't work that way. Grief that is colored by mixed emotions is more difficult. It is hard, when someone is gone, to admit to the negative feelings and harder yet to express them without feeling guilty. Counseling may be needed to sort out the mix of feelings accompanying this grief.

POSITIVE EFFECTS OF GRIEF

Grief can foster maturation. Sometimes, the death of someone dear leads the survivor to find new inner strength not obvious before.

> I recall a forty-year-old woman who had remained single and allowed her mother to make all her decisions throughout her life. They spoke daily, and the woman's grief following her mother's death was severe. After several months of exploring the loss in counseling sessions, and recognizing her need to depend on others, she began to rely more on herself and to become more confident of her own abilities. She continued to miss her mother, but as she adapted to the loss, she developed a stronger sense of herself and her potential as an independent and capable person.

Altruism can develop as a response to grief. Losing someone dear can lead to feelings of "I want to do something to honor his memory so people won't forget him." If the loss is of a child, the feeling may be "I want to be sure that no other child has to go through the illness my daughter did."

Finding a fitting memorial is a way of responding to grief. Gifts in memory of an individual who has died often go to an organization doing research on the disease that resulted in the person's death, such as the American Lung Association, the American Heart Association, and the American Cancer Society. Many foundations devoted to research in a particular disease come about because of grieving individuals who establish them in memory of the loved ones who died of cancer or AIDS, for example. The TJ Martell Foundation in New York, focusing on cancer, leukemia, and AIDS, was established by Tony and Vicki Martell, a father and mother who lost their twenty-one-year-old son, TJ, to leukemia. The foundation began as a way for these parents to honor their son and carry out his wishes that they help fight his disease by supporting research. The foundation has generously supported our work in exploring the human side of cancer.

Many of the volunteers at cancer centers or in hospices have lost someone precious; these survivors serve as volunteers because they "want to give back," to make it easier for someone else. Often they become volunteers in the very facility where the person died, so that they maintain a close relationship to the staff and a feeling of helping in a place where they understand the need.

MANAGEMENT OF NORMAL GRIEF

Studies of people going through grief show that the majority, about 80 percent, get through it with the help of their families, friends, and clergy. But 20 percent need some extra help, either one-on-one counseling or group support. Organizations spring up to meet the needs of specific groups. The Widow-to-Widow Program has been highly effective. Compassionate Friends has given help to many people who have lost their child. In Loving Memory, mentioned earlier in this chapter, helps parents who have lost their only child or all their children. Programs have also been started for children who have lost a parent to cancer or AIDS.

What helps to get through it? First, it is important to talk about it. The first thing grief counseling does is to encourage you to go over the details of the last days of illness, to talk about the sadness and the loss. People go over these details many times as they struggle to come to terms with what has happened to them. Talking with a sensitive listener is clearly helpful. This notion isn't exactly new. Shakespeare's Macbeth said, "Give Sorrow words, the grief that does not speak knits up the o'erwrought heart and bids it break."

Second, along with talking, it is important to express your emotions, such as sadness and loneliness. Crying and sobbing are okay; it's helpful to experience these feelings. People are embarrassed by crying in front of others and may work hard to keep their tears in check. Counseling allows and encourages this expression, which is part of the grief work, as you recall meaningful memories of places and times. Counseling can help you deal with the loss and to make sense of it in a way that enables you to go on.

Third, counseling, either individual or in a group, should be pursued if symptoms are severe or persistent. Many other resources exist nowadays to provide comfort: books, tapes, music, lectures. Most recently, the Internet has emerged as an unexpected resource, especially for people who are shy about talking face-to-face about their loss. Because the Internet has many people describing a range of experiences of loss, it is easier to find someone who truly "knows what you've been through." Remaining anonymous is a big plus for some (see Resources at the end of the book).

Children and adolescents who lose a parent often have trouble expressing their pain both to peers and to adults. They are anxious and depressed and frequently develop behavioral problems. Programs exist in many centers to help children and the healthy parent both before and after death. A program at Memorial called Kids' Express is run by social workers to help children cope with the loss of a parent. A similar one at New York Hospital, called

Kids' Net, is for children who have a parent with AIDS. These programs help to identify vulnerable children and parents. Several studies show that children whose surviving parent remains seriously depressed have more trouble. The support and care that the family receives after the loss is critically important in terms of adjustment in later life.

HOW GRIEF AFFECTS PHYSICAL HEALTH

Grief causes a profound disruption of biological rhythms. The hormonal and immune systems are affected, as evidenced by loss of sleep, appetite reduction, and weakness. Studies show a higher risk of death from suicide, accidents, cardiovascular disease, and some infectious diseases in survivors, especially men. However, studies show that women who have experienced a loss maintain a more healthy lifestyle than men who are left alone. This suggests that men should be more alert to their lifestyle and health concerns.

An important question often asked is whether grief increases risk of cancer or causes existing cancers to recur or progress.

I served on a panel appointed by the Institute of Medicine that carried out a major review of grief. We were surprised to find that the effects on mortality and vulnerability to disease were not as great as we had assumed. They appeared not to be of a magnitude to affect development of or recurrence of cancer. In a multicenter cancer clinical trials group (Cancer & Leukemia Group B), my colleagues and I confirmed these conclusions (see Chapter 3).

We have, in this chapter, discussed the nature of grief and suggested a number of ways that can help you with intense grieving. While many people handle grief well on their own, some have more difficulty in this struggle. Most people will benefit from using one or more of the sources of support that are available (see Resources). The good news is that the majority of people who grieve recover to go on with their lives; they may be altered and radically changed, but they do find a way to continue to face the future. And let's remember not to apply any time frame or outside expectations for this to happen; grief is a unique experience for each human being.

Our last thought as we leave you is that there are as many ways of grieving as there are ways of loving. The two are inextricably linked. Hold dear each of these many ways.

EPILOGUE

Writing *The Human Side of Cancer* has felt like an opportunity to share personally the experience of twenty years of talking with people as they coped with cancer, in the hope that what I have learned from them will be helpful to you. It has also provided an opportunity to try to sort out and make some sense out of the overwhelming amount of information extant in our society today about cancer and the emotions that accompany it—to try to clarify what relates to beliefs and attitudes and what comes from good clinical research. This "nonphysical" side of cancer is often neglected in the crunch of the physical aspects of cancer care, but I hope this book has confirmed for you that the "feeling" side of cancer is equally important and that the psychological, social, and spiritual aspects must be given equal attention.

Here are some of the take-home messages I would like to leave you with. First, you should take it with a grain of salt when someone tells you that you brought the cancer on yourself, or worse yet, that you "wanted the cancer" and that is why it developed. Our overzealous application of mind-body ideas can lead to "blaming the victim." I have come to the conclusion that believers in the mind-body connection are much like believers and nonbelievers in religion—you believe or you don't, and the facts and proof have little to do with it.

Another take-home message is that our society has led us to the belief that there is only one way to cope with cancer—by "positive thinking." I call it "the tyranny of positive thinking," because people who don't have it are badgered by family and well-meaning friends to get with it or they may contribute to a bad outcome from their cancer. There is no "one size fits all" way to cope. Our ways of coping are unique, like our fingerprints and our DNA—what we need is to respect and support each person's individual way of coping.

Imagining that one is the warrior on the white horse fighting cancer is great for some people, but it may be a disaster and an added burden for a quiet, self-contained person. Such a person told me, "If I have to be positive, I'll never make it. It just isn't me." So do whatever helps you cope and makes you feel better.

Coping with cancer is influenced by many things—our personalities, our prior experiences, especially with cancer, and the nature of the illness itself. Any one of these can make coping much harder. But just as people feel there is a stigma attached to cancer and want to keep it a secret, just as many others are embarrassed to ask for counseling and help in coping—experiencing the double fear of having cancer *and* being labeled as "mental" or "psychological" or, heaven forbid, "psychiatric." It is a sign of strength, not weakness, to ask help of people who are familiar with the psychological problems associated with cancer. Such help is available in most communities today. And there are many options for help, from groups to individual counseling to meditation, relaxation, and other behavioral interventions.

If *The Human Side of Cancer* has been able to ease the burden of your illness—or the illness of your loved one—even in a small way, then it has reached the goal with which I started the journey of this book—to make available what we have learned in twenty years of talking with people about their problems so that it can help others.

RESOURCES

GENERAL RESOURCES

American Cancer Society, Inc. (ACS), 1599 Clifton Road, NE, Atlanta, GA 30329, 800-ACS-2345 (website: www.cancer.org). Programs include Children's I I Camps, Hope Lodge, I Can Cope, Look Good . . . Feel Better, Man to Man, Reach to Recovery, Road to Recovery, and TLC. Dedicated to eliminating cancer as a major health problem through prevention, saving lives, and diminishing suffering, by means of research, education, advocacy, and service.

Association of Cancer Online Resources (website: www.acor.org). Online resources for cancer patients, caregivers, health professionals, and basic research scientists.

RJL Block Cancer Foundation, Inc. The Cancer Hotline, 4435 Main Street, Kansas City, MO 64111, 800-433-0464, 816-932-8453 (fax: 816-931-7486; e-mail: hotline@hrblock.com; websites: www.block.cancer.org, www.blast.cancer.org). Hotline matches newly diagnosed cancer patients with others who have survived the same kind of cancer. Offers free information, resources, and support groups, and distributes lists of multidisciplinary "second opinion centers." Also supplies three books at no charge: *Fighting Cancer, Cancer . . . There's Hope,* and *Guide for Cancer Supporters.*

Cancer Care, Inc., 275 Seventh Avenue, New York, NY 10001, 212-302-2400, 800-813-HOPE (fax: 212-719-0263; e-mail: info@cancercare.org; website: www.cancercare.org). Provides free professional counseling, support groups, education and information, and referrals to cancer patients and their families to help them cope with the psychological and social consequences of cancer.

Gilda's Club, 195 W. Houston Street, New York, NY 10014, 212-647-9700 (fax: 212-647-1151; website: www.gildasclub.org). A free, nonprofit program in which people with cancer and their families and friends join with others to build social and emotional support as a supplement to medical care in a nonresidential, homelike setting. Nineteen locations nationwide.

Look Good ... Feel Better, 1101 17th Street NW, Suite 300, Washington, DC 20036-4702, 1-800-395-LOOK (website: www.lgfb.org). This free public service program helps women undergoing treatment for cancer to overcome the possible physical side effects of receiving chemotherapy and/or radiation. The program is sponsored by the Cosmetic, Toiletry and Fragrance Association Foundation; The American Cancer Society; and the National Cosmetology Association.

MSKWeb (website: www.mskcc.org). Memorial Sloan-Kettering Cancer Center's website provides a wide range of information for medical professionals, patients, their families, and the general public.

National Cancer Institute (NCI). Cancer Information Service, 800-4-CANCER (fax 301-402-5874; website: www.nci.nih.gov). Provides a nationwide telephone service that answers questions and sends out booklets about cancer. Includes information about cancer treatment, screening, prevention, and supportive care.

Cancer Net. To get the Cancer Net contents list by e-mail, send an e-mail message that says "help" in the body of the message to cancernet@icicc.nci.nih.gov.

Cancer Trials (website: cancertrials.nci.nih.gov). This website provides up-to-date information on cancer clinical trials.

PDQ (Physician Data Query), 800-4-CANCER (website:www.nci.nih.gov). Computerized listing of up-to-date, accurate information on the latest types of cancer treatments, clinical trials, and organizations and doctors involved in caring for people with cancer.

National Comprehensive Cancer Network (NCCN), 800-ACS-2345, 888-909-NCCN (website: www.nccn.org). A coalition of eighteen comprehensive cancer centers has developed regularly updated guidelines for cancer treatment. Treatment guidelines available from numbers listed above as well as from *In-Touch Magazine*.

OncoLink. University of Pennsylvania Cancer Center, 3400 Spruce Street, 2 Donner, Philadelphia, PA 19104, 215-349-8895 (fax: 215-349-5445; e-mail: editors@oncolink.upenn.edu; website: www.oncolink.upenn.edu). Provides information about specific types of cancer, updates on cancer treatments, and news about research advances.

Vital Options TeleSupport Cancer Network. The Group Room Radio Talk Show, P.O. Box 19233, Encino, CA 91416-9233, 818-788-5225 (fax: 818-788-5260; website: www.vitaloptions.org). A weekly syndicated call-in cancer talk show linking callers with other patients, long-term survivors, family members, physicians, researchers, and therapists experienced in working with cancer issues.

The Wellness Community, 35 East 7th Street, Suite 412, Cincinnati, OH 45202, 888-793-WELL, 513-421-7111 (fax: 513-421-7119; e-mail: help@wellness-community.org; website: www.wellness-community.org).

Provides professionally led support groups nationwide and education, stress management, and social networking in a homelike community setting with a focus on enhancing health and well-being. Twenty facilities nationwide.

RESOURCES FOR PARTICULAR CANCERS

BRAIN TUMORS

American Brain Tumor Association, 2720 River Road, Suite 146, Des Plaines, IL 60018, 800-886-2282 (fax: 847-827-9918: e-mail: info@abta.org; website: www.abta.org). Offers free publications on brain tumors, social service consultations by telephone, a mentorship program, support group lists, a resource list of physicians, and a pen pal program. Also funds research nationwide.

The Brain Tumor Society, 124 Watertown Street, Suite 3-H, Watertown, MA 02472, 617-924-9997 (fax: 617-924-9998; e-mail: info@tbts.org; website: www.tbts.org). Provides individualized patient and family information, publishes educational materials, sponsors professional and patient conferences, and funds research.

National Brain Tumor Foundation, 785 Market Street, Suite 1600, San Francisco, CA 94103, 800-934-CURE, 415-284-0208 (fax: 415-284-0209; e-mail: nbtf@braintumor.org; website: www.braintumor.org). Raises funds for brain tumor research; provides support by offering contact with other brain tumor patients, information about treatment and local conferences, a listing of support groups, assistance starting support groups, and a newsletter.

BREAST CANCER

The Susan G. Komen Breast Cancer Foundation, 5005 LBJ Freeway, Suite 250, Dallas, TX 75244, 800-I'M AWARE (800-462-9273) (fax: 972-855-4301; e-mail: helpline@komen.org; website: www.breastcancer-info.com). Dedicated to eradicating breast cancer as a life-threatening disease by advancing research, education, screening, and treatment. Awards millions of dollars worth of grants and fellowships annually for groundbreaking breast cancer research.

National Alliance of Breast Cancer Organizations (NABCO), 9 East 37th Street, 10th Floor, New York, NY 10016, 888-80-NABCO (fax: 212-689-1213); e-mail: NABCOinfo@aol.com; website: www.nabco.org). A network of more than four hundred organizations that provide detection, treatment, and care to American women. Offers information, assistance, and referral to anyone with questions about breast cancer; educates the public about the disease; links underserved women to medical services; and acts as a voice for the interests and concerns of breast cancer survivors and women at risk.

National Breast Cancer Coalition, 1707 L Street NW, Suite 1060, Washington, DC 20036, 202-296-7477 (fax: 202-265-6854; website: www.stopbreastcancer.org). A grassroots advocacy organization whose goals are to increase federal funding for breast cancer research, influence how those dollars are spent, and improve access to high-quality health care for all women. Consists of more than five hundred member organizations and sixty thousand individual members throughout the United States.

National Lymphedema Network, Inc., 2211 Post Street, Suite 404, San Francisco CA 94115-3427, 415-921-1306, 800-541-3259 (fax: 415-921-4284; e-mail: nln@lymphnet.org; website: www.lymphnet.org). Publishes a quarterly newsletter, provides referrals, presents a biennial national conference, and offers educational materials for purchase.

SHARE Programs, 1501 Broadway, Suite 1720, New York, NY 10036, 212-719-0364 (website: www.sharecancersupport.org). Provides self-help programs for women with breast or ovarian cancer free of charge. Locations in New York City boroughs. Hotlines offer peer support in English and Spanish. Services include group support, wellness programs, Latina Share, education and advocacy efforts, and study of alternative/whole health issues.

Y-ME. National Breast Cancer Organization, 212 West Van Buren, Chicago, IL 60607, 800-221-2141 (24-hour), 800-986-9505 (24-hour Spanish) (fax: 312-294-8597; e-mail: help@y-me.org; website: www.y-me.org). Hotline counseling; educational programs; open-door meetings for breast cancer patients, their families, and friends; and a Y-ME Men's Support Line.

GASTROINTESTINAL CANCER

The Oley Foundation, 214 Hun Memorial, A-23, Albany Medical Center, Albany, NY 12208-3478, 518-262-5079 (fax: 518-262-5528; website: www.wizvax.net/oleyfdn). Provides free information and psychosocial support to patients fed by tube or IV at home who cannot be sustained by normal eating because part of their gastrointestinal tract is damaged or removed. However, it does not provide financial support or oral nutrition counseling.

United Ostomy Association. Inc., 19772 MacArthur Boulevard, Suite 200, Irvine, CA 92612-2405, 800-826-0826, 949-660-8624 (fax: 949-660-9262; e-mail: uoa@deltanet.com; website: www.uoa.org). Association of chapters dedicated to the complete rehabilitation of all ostomates.

GENITOURINARY CANCER

KIDNEY CANCER

Kidney Cancer Association, 1234 Sherman Avenue, Suite 203, Evanston, IL 60202-1375, 800-850-9132 (fax: 847-332-2978; e-mail: cdixon@NKCA.org; website: www.nkca.org). Works to increase the survival of kidney cancer patients and improve their care by providing information, sponsoring research, and acting as an advocate.

PROSTATE CANCER

American Foundation for Urologic Disease (AFUD), 1128 North Charles Street, Baltimore, MD 21201, 410-468-1800, 800-242-2383 (fax: 410-468-1808; e-mail: admin@afud.org; websites: http://www.afud.org and www.prostatehealth.com). Dedicated to the prevention and cure of urologic diseases through the expansion of research, education, awareness, and advocacy programs, including the Prostate Cancer Network.

Association for the Cure of Cancer of the Prostate (CaP CURE), 1250 4th Street, Suite 360, Santa Monica, CA 90401, 800-757-CURE; website: www.capcure.org).

Man-to-Man, 800-ACS-2345. Prostate cancer education and support program sponsored by the American Cancer Society. In some locations, Side by Side, a program for men with prostate cancer and their partners, is also available.

National Prostate Cancer Coalition, 1158 15th Street NW, Washington, DC 20005, 202-463-9455 (website: www.4npcc.org).

Patient Advocates for Advanced Cancer Treatments (PAACT), 1143 Parmelee NW, Grand Rapids, MI 49504, 616-453-1477 (fax: 616-453-1846; e-mail: pca@pcapaactinc.com; website: www.osz.com/paact). An association for both patients and physicians concerned with diagnostic methods and treatments of prostate cancer.

Us TOO International Inc. and **US TOO Partners (for spouses),** 930 North York Road, Suite 50, Hinsdale, IL 60521-2993, 800-808-7866, 630-323-1002 (fax: 630-323-1003; e-mail: ustoo@ustoo.com; website: www.ustoo.com). Support groups provide prostate cancer survivors and their families with emotional and educational support through a network of groups and a quarterly newsletter.

GYNECOLOGIC CANCER

National Ovarian Cancer Coalition, 2335 East Atlantic Boulevard, Suite 401, Pompano Beach, FL 33062, 888-0VARIAN, 954-781-3500 (fax: 954-781-3525; e-mail: NOCC@ovarian.com; website: www.ovarian.org). Raises awareness about ovarian cancer and promotes education regarding facts, issues, and problems.

The Ovarian Cancer Connection, P.O. Box 7948, Amarillo, TX 79114-7948, 806-355-2565 (fax: 806-467-9757; e-mail: chmelancon@aol.com; website: www.ovarian.news.com). Publishes *CONVERSATIONS! The Newsletter for Those Fighting Ovarian Cancer,* a monthly international newsletter providing hope, support, and information. Survivor-to-fighter matching service available.

Ovarian Cancer National Alliance, 1627 K Street NW, 12th Floor, Washington, DC 20006, 202-331-1332 (fax: 202-293-1990; e-mail: ovarian@aol.com; website: www.ovariancancer.org). A consumer-led umbrella organization dedicated to educating the public and the physicians who are likely to encounter the disease first about its symptoms, as well as advocating for more research, improved treatments, and a cure.

YWCA of the U.S.A. Office of Women's Health Initiatives, ENCOREplus Program, 624 9th Street NW, 3rd Floor, Washington, DC 20001-5303, 202-628-3636 (fax: 202-783-7123; e-mail: cgould@ywca.org; website: www.ywca.org). Targets medically underserved women in need of early detection, education, breast and cervical cancer screening, and support services.

LEUKEMIA

Leukemia and Lymphoma Society of America, 600 Third Avenue, New York, NY 10016, 800-955-4LSA (educational materials), 212-573-8484 (general information) (fax: 212-856-9686; website: www.leukemia.org). Dedicated to seeking the cause and eventual cure of leukemia and related cancers (lymphoma, Hodgkin's disease, and myeloma). Programs include research, patient aid, peer support, family support groups, and education.

LUNG CANCER

Alliance for Lung Cancer Advocacy, Support and Education (ALCASE), 1601 Lincoln Avenue, Vancouver, WA 98660, 800-298-2436 (fax: 360-699-1944; e-mail: info@alcase.org; website: www.alcase.org). Dedicated solely to helping people living with lung cancer. Programs are geared toward education about the disease, psychosocial support, and advocacy issues.

American Lung Association, 1740 Broadway, 14th Floor, New York, NY 10019-4374, 800-LUNG-USA, 212-315-8700 (fax: 212-265-5642; e-mail: info@lungusa.org; website: www.lungusa.org). Dedicated to preventing lung disease and promoting lung health.

LYMPHOMA

Cure for Lymphoma Foundation, 215 Lexington Avenue, New York, NY 10016, 800-CFL-6848, 212-213-9595 (fax: 212-213-9595; e-mail: infocfl@cfl.org; website: www.cfl.org). Funds lymphoma research. Provides support and educational materials via quarterly newsletter, informational booklets, fact sheet, and comprehensive lymphoma library.

Lymphoma Research Foundation of America, Inc., 8800 Venice Boulevard, #207, Los Angeles, CA 90034, 310-204-7040 (fax: 310-204-7043; e-mail: LRFA@aol.com; website: www.lymphoma.org). Funds lymphoma research and provides information and emotional support to patients and caregivers through educational materials, the Lymphoma Helpline, the national Cell-Mates buddy program linking patients, a quarterly newsletter, support groups, an annual patient educational forum, and local seminars. Sponsors National Lymphoma Awareness Week, Lymphoma Advocacy Day, and an annual Lymphoma Think Tank.

MULTIPLE MYELOMA

International Myeloma Foundation, 2129 Stanley Hills Drive, Los Angeles, CA 90046, 800-452-CURE (fax: 323-656-1182; e-mail: TheIMF@aol.com; website: www.myeloma.org). Promotes education, funds research, holds patient and family seminars and clinical and scientific conferences. Publishes a quarterly newsletter, *Myeloma Today*.

Multiple Myeloma Research Foundation (MMRF), 11 Forest Street, New Canaan, CT 06840, 203-972-1250 (fax: 203-972-1259; website: www.multiplemyeloma.org). Supports research and professional symposia on multiple myeloma and related cancers. Publishes a quarterly newsletter and provides referrals and information to patients and family members.

OTHER RESOURCES

AGING

U.S. Administration on Aging (website: aoa.dhhs.gov). Information for older persons, families, practitioners, researchers, students, and the aging network.

The American Geriatrics Society (website: www.americangeriatrics.org). Links to AGS publications, selected bibliography, consumer education, related news.

ALTERNATIVE AND COMPLEMENTARY THERAPIES

Bibliographic Summary of Information (website: cpmcnet.columbia.edu/dept/rosenthal/databases/AM_databases.html).

NIH Office of Alternative Medicine Citation Index (website: altmed.od.nih.gov/oam/resources/cam-ci).

University of Texas Center for Alternative Medicine Research in Cancer (website: chprd.sph.uth.tmc.edu/utcam).

Bone Marrow Transplantation

Blood & Marrow Transplant (BMT) Newsletter, 2900 Skokie Valley Road, Highland Park, IL 60035, 847-433-3313, 888-597-5674 (fax: 847-433-4599; e-mail: help@bmtnews.org; website: www.bmtnews.org). Publishes a quarterly newsletter and a book for bone marrow, peripheral stem cell, and cord blood transplant patients. Offers an attorney list to help resolve insurance problems, as well as a "patient-to-survivor telephone link."

National Bone Marrow Transplant Link (NBMT Link), 29209 Northwestern Highway, #624, Southfield, MI 48034, 800-LINK-BMT (fax: 248-932-8483; website: comnet.org/nbmtlink). Provides peer support to BMT patients and their families. Serves as an information center for prospective BMT patients and health professionals. NBMT Link offers three educational publications.

National Marrow Donor Program, 3433 Broadway Street NE, Suite 500, Minneapolis, MN 55413, 800-MARROW-2 (fax: 612-627-8125; website: www.marrow.org). Network maintains a data bank of available tissue-typed marrow donor volunteers nationwide. Program provides information and support to patients in search of an unrelated marrow donor.

Caregivers

Caregiver Network (website: www.caregiver.on.ca:80/index.html). Canadian-based; bulletin board, links, and support for caregivers.

Family Caregiver Alliance, 690 Market Street, Suite 600, San Francisco, CA 94104, 415-434-3388 (fax: 415-434-3508; e-mail: info@caregiver.org; website: www.caregiver.org). Help for caregivers, featuring support groups and resource guide for families coping with cancer and other disorders.

Well Spouse Foundation, 30 East 40 Street, New York, NY 10016, 212-685-8815, 800-838-0879 (fax: 212-685-8676; e-mail: wellspouse@aol.com). Association of spousal caregivers.

Children

Candlelighters Childhood Cancer Foundation, 7910 Woodmont Avenue, Suite 460, Bethesda, MD 20814-3015, 301-657-8401, 800-366-2223 (fax: 301-718-2686; e-mail: info@candlelighters.org; websites: www.candlelighters.org and www.candle.org). Provides information, support, and advocacy to families of children with cancer, survivors of childhood cancer, and professionals who work with them.

Children Coping with Grief and Dying (website: www.Grannyg.bc.ca/ckidbook.grief.html). Books dealing with aspects of grief and loss from the perspective of children. Collected by Lee Anne Phillips. Provides brief description of each book, but no ordering from site.

Friends Network, P.O. Box 4545, Santa Barbara, CA 93140 (phone and fax: 805-693-1017; website: www.cancerfunletter.com). Offers a cancer activities bimonthly newsletter *(Funletter)* for kids and additional support for patients and families.

Kids Konnected, 27071 Cabot Road, Suite 102, Laguna Hills, CA 92653, 800-899-2866, 949-582-5443 (fax: 949-582-3989; e-mail: JWH@kids-konnected.org; website: www.kidskonnected.org). Provides friendship, education, understanding, and support to kids who have a parent with cancer.

National Childhood Cancer Foundation (NCCF), 440 East Huntington, P.O. Box 60012, Arcadia, CA 91066-6012, 626-447-1674, 800-458-6223 (website: www.nccf.org). Supports nationwide clinical and laboratory research on causes, treatments, and cures for childhood cancer, and advocates to benefit children with cancer.

Pediatric Pain Research Laboratory (website: is.dal.ca/~pedpain). Affiliated with Dalhousie University, Halifax, Nova Scotia, Canada. Provides professional research and self-help resources related to children in pain.

Ronald McDonald House, Ronald McDonald House Charities, One Kroc Drive, Oak Brook, IL 60523, 630-623-7048 (fax: 630-623-7488; website: www.rmhc.com). Offers a refuge from the hospital, a "home-away-from-home."

NEWSLETTERS AND MAGAZINES

Coping with Cancer, P.O. Box 682268, Franklin, TN 37068-2268, 615-790-2400 (fax: 615-794-0179; e-mail: copingmag@aol.com). Consumer magazine for people whose lives have been touched by cancer. Provides knowledge, hope, and inspiration from cancer survivors and health care professionals. Provides official annual coverage of National Cancer Survivors Day and is a national sponsor.

International Cancer Alliance (ICA), 4853 Cordell Avenue, Suite 11, Bethesda, MD 2081, 800-I CARE-61 (fax: 301-654-8684; e-mail: sysent@ari.net; website: www.icare.org). Provides a free cancer therapy review, which includes information on a specific type of cancer (description, detection and staging, treatment, and clinical trials). *Cancer Breakthroughs* (a newsletter) is sent quarterly.

Melanoma Update, Memorial Sloan-Kettering Cancer Center, Box 421, 1275 York Avenue, New York, NY 10021. A free newsletter for melanoma patients and their families. Excerpts news articles about melanoma and provides commentary on the information by professionals working in melanoma. Published twice a year.

The Sarcoma Newsletter, Department of Social Work, MSKCC, 1275 York
Avenue, New York, NY 10021. Provides patients with important information about the disease, treatment, side effects, resources for information, places to help, and stories from survivors.

PAIN MANAGEMENT

Resource Center for State Cancer Pain Initiative (website:
www.wisc.edu/molpharm/wcpi). Provides an advocacy network concerning cancer pain.

Roxane Pain Institute (website: www.Roxane.com/Roxane/PRI).
Cancer and AIDS pain management educational materials. Downloadable
pain management slide show, dates of lectures/seminars, and links to
patient and professional "libraries."

PALLIATIVE/HOSPICE CARE, GRIEF, AND BEREAVEMENT

Bereavement and Hospice Support Netline (websites: www.ubalt.edu
and www.bereavement). Public service on-line directory of bereavement
support groups.

Choice in Dying, 1035 30th Street NW, Washington, DC 20007, 800-
989-WILL, 202-338-9790 (fax: 202-338-0242; e-mail: cid@choices.org;
website: www.choices.org). Advocates recognition and protection of individual rights at the end of life. Provides counseling regarding preparing
and using living wills and durable powers of attorney for health care.

Dying Well (website: www.dyingwell.com). Resources for patients and
families facing life-limiting illness.

The End of Life: Exploring Death in America (website:
www.npr.org/programs/death). National Public Radio's transcripts of
programs in its ongoing series about death and dying in America, available with a resource guide and personal stories posted by site visitors.
Selections from novels and short stories, poems, religious rituals, clinical
research, scripts for plays and television, and radio programs.

Grief Net (website: www.griefnet.org). A system that connects to a variety
of resources related to death, dying, bereavement, and major emotional
and physical losses. Offers information as well as discussion/support
groups. Has a section for children as well.

Make Today Count, c/o Connie Zimmerman, St. John's Mid-America
Cancer Center, 1235 E. Cherokee, Springfield, MO 65804-2263, 800-
432-2273 (fax: 417-888-8761). A mutual support organization that brings
together persons affected by a life-threatening illness so they may help
each other.

National Hospice Organization (NHO), 1901 North Moore Street,
Suite 901, Arlington, VA 22209, 703-243-5900, 800-658-8898 (fax: 703-

525-5762; e-mail: drsnho@cais.com; website: www.nho.org). Hospice Helpline helps callers find a hospice in their area.

PREVENTION

American Institute for Cancer Research (AICR), 1759 R Street NW, Washington, DC 20009, 800-843-8114, 202-328-7744 (fax: 202-328-7226; website: www.aicr.org). Focuses on the link between diet and cancer, supports research in this field nationwide, and provides a wide range of free educational publications.

SURVIVORS

National Cancer Survivors Day (NCSD) Foundation, P.O. Box 682285, Franklin, TN 37068-2285, 615-794-3006 (fax: 615-794-0179; e-mail: ncsd@aol.com; website: www.ncsdf.org). NCSD is the world's largest cancer survivor event and is celebrated on the first Sunday in June of each year in more than seven hundred communities throughout North America. A free celebration planning kit is available from the foundation.

National Coalition for Cancer Survivorship (NCCS), 1010 Wayne Avenue, Silver Spring, MD 20910, 888-650-9127 (fax: 301-565-9670; e-mail: info@cansearch.org; website: www.cansearch.org). The only patient-led organization advocating on behalf of survivors of all types of cancer. NCCS's mission is to lead and strengthen the survivorship movement, empower cancer survivors, and advocate for policy issues that affect cancer survivors' quality of life.

The Park Ridge Center (website: www.Prchfe.org/publications/bulletin/7.html). The center's bulletin focuses on spirituality in health care.

Patient Advocate Foundation (PAF), 780 Pilot House Drive, Suite 100C, Newport News, VA 23606, 800-532-5274, 757-873-6668 (fax: 757-873-8999; website: www.patientadvocate.org). Provides patient education relative to managed-care terminology and policy issues that may affect coverage, legal intervention services, and counseling to resolve job and insurance problems.

TRANSPORTATION

Corporate Angel Network, Inc. (CAN), One Loop Road, Westchester County Airport, White Plains, NY 10604, 914-328-1313 (website: www.corpangelnetwork.org). Provides free plane transportation for cancer patients going to and from recognized cancer treatment centers by using empty seats aboard corporate aircraft operating on business flights. There are no financial requirements or limits on number of trips.

National Patient Air Transport Helpline (NPATH), P.O. Box 1940, Manassas, VA 20108-0804, 800-296-1217 (fax: 757-318-9107; e-mail:

npathmsg@aol.com; website: www.npath.org). Makes referrals to charitable and special discounted patient medical air transport services, based on an evaluation of patients' needs.

WOMEN

Mautner Project for Lesbians with Cancer, 1707 I Street NW, Suite 500, Washington, DC 20036, 202-332-5536 (fax: 202-332-0662; e-mail: mautner@mautnerproject.org; website: http://www.mautnerproject.org). Provides support, education, information, and advocacy for health issues relating to lesbians with cancer, their partners, and their families.

National Women's Health Information Center, Office of Women's Health, U.S. Department of Health and Human Services, Washington, DC. Provides access to women's health information from the federal government and the private sector.

BOOKS FOR ADULTS

ALTERNATIVE AND COMPLEMENTARY THERAPIES

Cassileth, B. R. *The Alternative Medicine Handbook: The Complete Reference Guide to Alternative and Complementary Therapies.* New York: W.W. Norton & Company, 1998.

Fetrow, C. W., and Avila, J. R. *Complementary and Alternative Medicines.* Springhouse, PA: Springhouse, 1999.

Lerner, M.: *Choices in Healing.* Cambridge, MA: MIT Press, 1996.

BEREAVEMENT AND GRIEF

Baugher, R., and Calija, M. *A Guide for the Bereaved Survivor: A List of Reactions, Suggestions, and Steps for Coping with Grief.* Renton, WA: Robert Baugher, 1993.

Bernstein, J. R. *When the Bough Breaks: Forever After the Death of a Son or Daughter.* Kansas City, MO: Andrews McMeel Publishing, 1998.

Blank, J. W. *The Death of an Adult Child: A Book for and About Bereaved Parents.* Amityville, NY: Baywood Publishing Company, 1998.

Fitzgerald, H. *The Grieving Child: A Parent's Guide.* New York: Simon & Schuster, 1992.

Kübler-Ross, E. *On Death and Dying.* New York: Simon & Schuster, 1997.

Lewis, C. S. *A Grief Observed.* New York: HarperCollins, 1989.

Rando, T. A. *Grieving: How to Go on Living When Someone You Love Dies.* Lexington, MA: Lexington Books, 1988.

COPING

Block, R., and Block, A. *Fighting Cancer*. Kansas City, MO: R.A. Block Cancer Foundation, 1992.

Cousins, N. *Anatomy of an Illness Perceived by the Patient: Reflections on Healing and Regeneration*. New York: Bantam, Doubleday, Dell Publishers, 1991.

Fiore, N. *The Road Back to Health: Coping with the Emotional Aspects of Cancer*. New York: Bantam, Doubleday, Dell Publishers, 1984.

Harpham, W. S. *Diagnosis: Cancer—Your Guide Through the First Few Months*. New York: W.W. Norton & Company, 1998.

———. *When a Parent Has Cancer: A Guide to Caring for Your Children*. New York: HarperCollins, 1997.

Larschan, E. J., and Larschan, R. J. *The Diagnosis Is Cancer: A Psychological and Legal Resource Handbook for Cancer Patients, Their Families and Helping Professionals*. New York: Bull Publishing Company, 1986.

Lipsyte, R. *In the Country of Illness: Comfort and Advice for the Journey*. New York: Alfred A. Knopf, 1998.

Love, S. *Dr. Susan Love's Breast Book*. New York: Perseus Press, 1995.

Pennebaker, J. W. *Opening Up: The Healing Power of Expressing Emotions*. New York: Guilford Press, 1990.

Price, R. *A Whole New Life: An Illness and a Healing*. New York: Penguin Books, 1995.

Radner, G. *It's Always Something*. New York: Avon Books, 1995.

Roloff, A. T. *Navigating Through a Strange Land: A Book for Brain Tumor Patients and Their Families*. Sheffield, MA: Option Indigo Press, 1995.

Schimmel, S. R., and Fox, B. *Cancer Talk: Voices of Hope and Endurance from "The Group Room," the World's Largest Cancer Support Group*. New York: Broadway Books, 1999.

HUMOR

Wicks, B. *Ben Wicks on Ovarian Cancer: The Disease That Whispers*. Toronto, Canada: Ben Wicks & Associates, 1998.

———. *Ben Wicks' So You've Got Cancer*. Toronto, Canada: Ben Wicks & Associates, 1997.

MEANING AND SPIRITUALITY

Bedard, J. *Lotus in the Fire: The Healing Power of Zen*. Boston: Shambhala Publications, 1999.

Canfield, J., and Hansen, M. V. *Chicken Soup for the Soul: 101 Stories to Open the Heart and Rekindle the Spirit*. Deerfield Beach, FL: Health Communications, 1996.

Coles, R. *The Call of the Stories: Teaching and the Moral Imagination*. New York: Houghton Mifflin Co., 1990.

Frankl, V. E. *Man's Search for Meaning*. New York: Washington Square Press, 1984.

Kabat-Zinn, J. *Wherever You Go, There You Are*. New York: Hyperion Press, 1995.

Kübler-Ross, E. *The Wheel of Life*. New York: Scribner, 1997.

Kushner, H. S. *When Bad Things Happen to Good People*. New York, Avon Books, 1981.

MEDICINE AND SOCIETY

Rothman, D. *Strangers at the Bedside: A History of How Law and Bioethics Transformed Medical Decision Making*. New York: Basic Books, 1991.

PALLIATIVE AND TERMINAL CARE

Callahan, D. *The Troubled Dream of Life: In Search of a Peaceful Death*. New York: Simon & Schuster, 1993.

PERSONAL ACCOUNTS

Albom, M. *Tuesdays with Morrie: An Old Man, a Young Man, and Life's Greatest Lesson*. New York: Doubleday, 1997.

Conway, K. *Ordinary Life, A Memoir of Illness*. New York: W.H. Freeman & Company, 1997.

Groopman, J. *The Measure of Our Days: New Beginnings at Life's End*. New York: Viking Press, 1997.

Ryan, C., and Ryan, K. M. *A Private Battle*. New York: Fawcett Popular Library, 1980.

Sontag, S. *Illness as Metaphor and AIDS and Its Metaphors*. New York: Doubleday, 1990.

Spingarn, N. *The New Cancer Survivors: Living with Grace, Fighting with Spirit*. Baltimore, MD: Johns Hopkins University Press, 1999.

Williams, T. T. *Refuge: An Unnatural History of Family and Place*. New York: Vantage Books, 1992.

Winawer, S. J., and Taylor N. *Healing Lessons*. Boston: Little, Brown & Co., 1998.

PREVENTION

Winawer, S. J., Shike, M., Bashe, P., and Subak-Sharpe, G. *Cancer Free*. New York, Simon & Schuster, 1995.

SEXUALITY

Schover, L. R. *Sexuality and Cancer: For the Man Who Has Cancer and His Partner.* Atlanta, GA: American Cancer Society, 1988.

———. *Sexuality and Cancer: For the Woman Who Has Cancer and Her Partner.* Atlanta, GA: American Cancer Society, 1988.

———. *Sexuality and Fertility After Cancer.* New York: John Wiley & Sons, 1997.

SURVIVORS

Armstrong, L. *It's Not About the Bike: My Journey Back to Life.* New York: Putnam, 2000.

U.S. Department of Health and Human Services. *Facing Forward: A Guide for Cancer Survivors.* Bethesda, MD: National Institutes of Health, 1990.

———

FOR YOUNG READERS

Brisson, P. *Sky Memories.* New York: Random House, 1999.

Buscaglia, L. *The Fall of Freddie the Leaf.* New York: Holt, Rinehart & Winston, 1983.

Tiffault, B. W. *A Quilt for Elizabeth.* Burnsville, NC: Rainbow Connection, 1992.

Trillin, A. *Dear Bruno.* New York: The New Press, 1996.

Weil, K. *Zink the Zebra.* Milwaukee: Gareth Stevens Publishing, 1996.

Williams, M. *The Velveteen Rabbit.* New York: Derrydale Books, 1986.

INDEX

Q & A with Jimmie Holland, M.D.

Q: As a psychiatrist, how did you come to work with people with cancer?

A: I have always been interested not only in people's medical problems but also in how they adjusted to them, how they got on with their lives. Years ago in the 1950s I was listening to my husband, Jim, an oncologist who did early investigations in chemotherapy for leukemia, and his colleagues discuss the side effects of chemotherapy and other treatments that were new at the time. But when I asked, "How do the patients *feel* about the treatments?" I was met with blank stares. At that time, the focus was on changing the bleak survival statistics. There was little thought about what it meant emotionally to be diagnosed with cancer, to get sick from the chemotherapy, and to be frightened that the cancer might come back and that you might not survive.

I began to talk to people with cancer and to study their responses to hearing their diagnosis or to finishing a course of treatment. In one of my earliest studies, we learned that women completing their radiation treatment for breast cancer had *more* distress at the *end* of treatment. We found that they felt fearful when the treatment stopped because the tumor could come back and they missed seeing the doctor and staff every day, which made them feel more secure. They feared being on their own.

Q: Are most people with cancer depressed?

A: No, but many do experience *distress*: being fearful, worried, and sad is normal when you confront a threat to your life. But the normal level of distress can become greater and may reach the level of depression or severe anxiety. Both normal and abnormal levels of distress can be helped by talking to a counselor, by meditating, or if needed, by taking medication. Unfortunately, most doctors don't ask their cancer patients if they are having distress—they tend to focus mainly on the "medical" side of cancer. Just as unfortunately, most patients don't volunteer the information. They're afraid that the doctor will think they're a wimp or that they'll be a burden to their family and friends, so they keep it to themselves. This "don't ask, don't tell" situation doesn't help anyone.

It's important to realize that everyone has down days—that's a normal part of being ill. But if you're unable to function normally—if you can't get out of bed in the morning, can't eat, or can't sleep at night—then you need to tell your doctor so that you can get the support you need to go on.

Q: What would you recommend to someone who is having a hard time coping?

A: There is so much help available today, and it comes in many forms. That's why we call the chapter about different psychological therapies "All Medicine Doesn't Come in a Bottle." For example, different forms of counseling can assist people with cancer and their family members in coping: individual counseling, group counseling, self-help groups (led by peers). Scientific studies have also shown that techniques you can practice by yourself, or with a family member or friend, such as a relaxation exercise or guided imagery, can relieve the burden of your illness and help you cope better. This book includes a number of these exercises and techniques.

Q: What kind of help do family members need?

A: It's very hard to watch someone you love go through a challenging course of treatment and to worry whether she or he will survive. Loved ones have the additional burden of taking over other responsibilities, such as taking care of the kids, home, finances, insurance matters, as well as giving physical and emotional support to the one who is ill. Families have a far greater burden today when patients are discharged from the hospital "sicker and quicker," and more care falls on the family to manage. Individual, family, and group counseling for loved ones is available in many communities.

There are also groups for children of cancer patients as well as bereavement counseling or support groups that can be very healing.

Q: You have mentioned myths based on social attitudes about cancer. What are they?

A: The first is that cancer equals death, which is no longer true. There are 8 million cancer survivors in the United States. There are new treatments all the time. Many people will experience a complete recovery; others may have cancer as a chronic illness, like prostate cancer.

Another myth is the notion that some flaw in your character—or your personality—causes cancer. Yet another is this belief that you have to maintain a positive attitude twenty-four hours a day, seven days a week, to prevent your illness from progressing. In the book we call this "the Tyranny of Positive Thinking." To my mind, the research on all of these points does not demonstrate that we bring cancer on ourselves or worsen our chances for survival through our personality, emotions, attitudes, or the stress we experience in life.

Q: Dr. Holland, how did you come to write *The Human Side of Cancer?*

A: Over the more than twenty years I have been working with people with cancer and their loved ones, many have asked me to recommend a book to help them cope. Unfortunately, many of the books out there today say you have to cope in one particular way, suggesting that to regain health and do well, you need to keep a positive attitude, attend a support group, or follow another specific approach. This just isn't so. Many people are helped by each of these practices, but there is no one-size-fits-all way of coping. There are many different ways that work, and we should respect each individual's unique way of coping as we respect other personal differences.

The initial impulse behind this book was to give people a kind of road map of the cancer journey. What is it like for most people to face a cancer diagnosis, to go through a challenging course of treatment, to cope with the uncertainty that cancer brings into a person's life? What kind of help is available to you if your natural way of coping *isn't* working for you? These are among the many questions we wanted to answer.

To help make the book more user-friendly, I asked Sheldon Lewis, a journalist interested in psychological aspects of health as well as complementary approaches people can do for themselves, such as meditation, relaxation, and guided imagery, to work with me.